W9-BNX-040

Computer Simulation and Experimental Assessment of Cardiac Electrophysiology

Edited by

Nathalie Virag, PhD
Olivier Blanc, MS
Lukas Kappenberger, MD

Lausanne, Switzerland

Futura Publishing Company, Inc.
Armonk, NY

FUTURA

Library of Congress Cataloging-in-Publication Data

Computer simulation and experimental assessment of cardiac electrophysiology / edited by Nathalie Virag, Lukas Kappenberger, Olivier Blanc.
    p. ; cm.
  Papers from the Second International Workshop on Computer Simulation and Experimental Assessment of Electrical Cardiac Function, held Dec. 4–5, 2000 in Lausanne, Switzerland.
  Includes bibliographical references and index.
  ISBN 0-87993-492-1 (alk. paper)
    1. Arrhythmia—Computer simulation—Congresses. 2. Heart—Contraction—Computer simulation—Congresses. I. Virag, Nathalie. II. Kappenberger, Lukas. III. Blanc, Olivier, MS. IV. International Workshop on Computer Simulation and Experimental Assessment of Electrical Cardiac Function (2nd : 2000 : Lausanne, Switzerland)
  [DNLM: 1. Arrhythmia—diagnosis—Congresses. 2. Electrophysiologic Techniques, Cardiac—Congresses. 3. Arrhythmias—therapy—Congresses. 4. Computer Simulation—Congresses. WG 330 C738 2001]
  RC685.A65 C565 2001
  616.1'28—dc21

                                        2001033459

Copyright © 2001
Futura Publishing Company, Inc.
135 Bedford Road
Armonk, New York 10504
www.futuraco.com

ISBN #:0-87993-492-1

Printed in the United States of America on acid-free paper.

Contributors

Maurits Allessie, MD, PhD   Professor and Chairman, Department of Physiology, University of Maastricht, Maastricht, The Netherlands

Jacques Beaumont, PhD   Assistant Professor, Department of Pharmacology, SUNY Upstate Medical University, Syracuse, NY

Olivier Blanc, MS   Signal Processing Laboratory, Swiss Federal Institute of Technology, Lausanne, Switzerland

Nipon Chattipakorn, MD, PhD   Division of Cardiovascular Disease, Department of Medicine, The University of Alabama, Birmingham, AL

Piero Colli-Franzone, PhD   Professor, Department of Mathematics and Institute of Numerical Analysis, University of Pavia, Pavia, Italy

Nastasja M.S. de Groot, MD   Department of Physiology, Cardiovascular Research Institute Maastricht, University of Maastricht, Maastricht, The Netherlands

Igor Efimov, PhD   Elmer L. Lindseth Associate Professor of Biomedical Engineering, Case Western Reserve University, Cleveland, OH

Olaf Eick, PhD   Bakken Research Center, Maastricht, The Netherlands

Martin Fromer, MD   Division of Cardiology, Centre Hospitalier Universitaire Vaudois, Lausanne, Switzerland

David M. Harrild, PhD   Department of Biomedical Engineering, Duke University, Durham, NC

Craig S. Henriquez, PhD   Associate Professor, Department of Biomedical Engineering, Duke University, Durham, NC

Hanspeter Herzel, PhD   Professor, Institute for Theoretical Biology, Humbold University, Berlin, Germany

Siew Y. Ho, PhD, FRCPath   Reader in Cardiac Morphology, National Heart & Lung Institute, Imperial College, London, UK

Peter J. Hunter, PhD   Professor, Department of Engineering Science, University of Auckland, New Zealand

Raymond E. Ideker, MD, PhD   Professor, Division of Cardiovascular Disease, Department of Medicine, The University of Alabama, Birmingham, AL

Vincent Jacquemet, MS   Signal Processing Laboratory, Swiss Federal Institute of Technology, Lausanne, Switzerland

José Jalife, MD   Professor and Chairman of Pharmacology, Professor of Medicine and Pediatrics, SUNY Upstate Medical University, Syracuse, NY

Lukas Kappenberger, MD   Professor and Chairman, Division of Cardiology, Centre Hospitalier Universitaire Vaudois, Lausanne, Switzerland

Jacques Koerfer, MD   Division of Cardiology, Centre Hospitalier Universitaire Vaudois, Lausanne, Switzerland

Andrew D. McCulloch, PhD   Professor, Department of Bioengineering, Whitaker Institute for Biomedical Engineering, University of California, San Diego, La Jolla, CA

Elliot McVeigh, PhD   Laboratory of Cardiac Energetics, National Heart Lung and Blood Institute, National Institutes of Health, Bethesda, MD

Anushka Michailova, MS   Department of Bioengineering, Whitaker Institute for Biomedical Engineering, University of California, San Diego, La Jolla, CA

Peter J. Mulquiney, PhD   Department of Biochemistry, Oxford University, UK

Denis Noble, PhD, FRS, Hon FRCP   Professor, University Laboratory of Physiology, Oxford University, UK

S. Bertil Olsson, MD, PhD   Professor, Department of Cardiology, University Hospital, Lund, Sweden

Alexandre Panfilov, PhD   University Docent, Department of Theoretical Biology, Utrecht University, The Netherlands

Arkady M. Pertsov, PhD   Associated Professor, Department of Pharmacology, SUNY Upstate Medical University, Syracuse, NY

Etienne Pruvot, MD   Division of Cardiology, Centre Hospitalier Universitaire Vaudois, Lausanne, Switzerland

Yoram Rudy, PhD   Professor of Biomedical Engineering, Physiology & Biophysics, and Medicine, Director, Cardiac Bioelectricity Center, Case Western University, Cleveland, OH

Frank B. Sachse, PhD   Institute of Biomedical Engineering, University of Karlsruhe (TH), Karlsruhe, Germany

Faramarz H. Samie, PhD   Department of Pharmacology, SUNY Upstate Medical University, Syracuse, NY

Gunnar Seemann, MS   Institute of Biomedical Engineering, University of Karlsruhe (TH), Karlsruhe, Germany

Nicolas P. Smith, PhD   University Laboratory of Physiology, Oxford University, UK

Derrick Sung, MS   Department of Bioengineering, Whitaker Institute for Biomedical Engineering, University of California, San Diego, La Jolla, CA

Mary Ellen Thomas, MS   Department of Bioengineering, Whitaker Institute for Biomedical Engineering, University of California, San Diego, La Jolla, CA

Natalia A. Trayanova, Ph.D   Associate Professor, Department of Biomedical Engineering, Tulane University, New Orleans, LA

Jean-Marc Vesin, PhD   Signal Processing Laboratory, Swiss Federal Institute of Technology, Lausanne, Switzerland

Nathalie Virag, PhD   Lausanne, Switzerland

Albert L. Waldo, MD   The Walter H. Pritchard Professor of Cardiology and Professor of Medicine, Division of Cardiology, University Hospitals of Cleveland, Cleveland, OH

Christian D. Werner, MS   Institute of Biomedical Engineering, University of Karlsruhe (TH), Karlsruhe, Germany

Christian Zemlin, MS   Institute for Theoretical Biology, Humbold University, Berlin, Germany

Preface

Computer modeling is a rapidly growing field that promotes interactions between scientists from different horizons such as engineers, mathematicians, basic electrophysiologists and clinicians.

The purpose of this book is to spread a constructive spirit of collaboration in the field of computer modeling and this book covers a wide variety of topics. The two first parts show how computer modeling of electrical propagation and electrical mapping of the atria and the ventricles respectively can contribute to our understanding of arrhythmias in humans. The third part covers the aspect of computer modeling of mechanical contractions of the heart. In the fourth part, we can see how, as computation power increases, we can design computer models of the whole heart that are more and more realistic. Finally, the last two parts describe the therapeutic strategies for atrial and ventricular arrhythmias respectively. They also show how computer simulations can be used as a tool to test therapeutic strategies.

Despite all this enthusiasm the critical question remains: Is computer modeling useful for the development of new therapeutic strategies? We hope that this book contributes to answer this crucial question by providing an overview on what can be done today in this area.

We would like to express our gratitude to all the authors who accepted to contribute to this book with extremely interesting manuscripts. This would not have been possible without a grant from the Collomed Foundation in Lausanne, Switzerland. We also would like to thank Futura Publishing for working at such short notice and the Theo Rossi di Montelera Foundation for their continuous support of innovative research.

Nathalie Virag
Olivier Blanc
Lukas Kappenberger

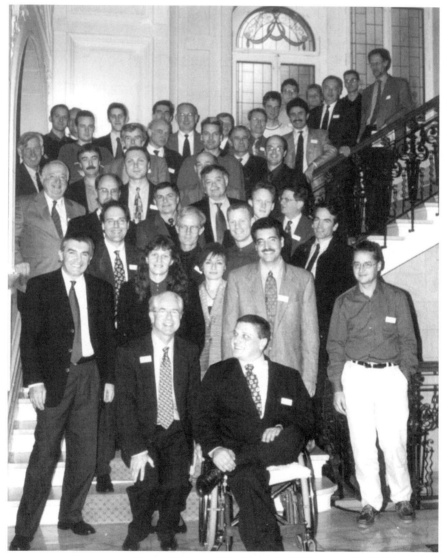

Group Picture of the Contributors.

Dedication

In Memory of Conte Theo Rossi di Montelera who, with his humanistic spirit, stimulated the concept of union between basic science and bedside medicine.

Contents

Part I.

Electrical Mapping and Modeling of Atria

Chapter 1

Ten Years of Mapping of Human Atrial Fibrillation

Natasja M.S. de Groot, MD,
Maurits Allessie, MD, PhD

Introduction

Cardiac mapping has been defined as: "A method by which cardiac signals are recorded from multiple sites of the heart and spatially depicted as a function of time in an integrated manner."[1] It requires determination of the local activation time at each electrode and the creation of activation maps which provide a spatial model of the activation sequence. In general, mapping can be used to elucidate the mechanism of arrhythmias and to guide therapy. With respect to atrial fibrillation (AF), mapping is useful to analyse intra-atrial conduction patterns and to diagnose the electro-anatomical substrate. Knowledge of the mechanisms underlying AF can provide a basis for development of innovative therapies. Examples of such new therapies of AF are focal ablation of the origin of ectopic beats,[2,3] isolation of the pulmonary veins,[4] and the creation of linear lesions either by surgical incisions or radiofrequency catheter ablation.[5-7]

In this review, we will limit ourselves to mapping of human AF. Although the number of human mapping studies is still rather limited, it is useful to discuss *induced* and *chronic* AF separately.

Induced Atrial Fibrillation

The first mapping study of human AF was performed in 1991 by Cox et al. in patients with the Wolff-Parkinson White syndrome undergoing cardiac surgery for interruption of their accessory atrio-ventricular path-

From Virag N, Blanc O, Kappenberger L (eds): *Computer Simulation and Experimental Assessment of Cardiac Electrophysiology.* ©Futura Publishing Co., Inc., Armonk, NY, 2001.

way.[8] AF was induced by burst-pacing and both the right and left atria were mapped using epicardial templates (160 bipolar electrodes, interelectrode distance 5–10 mm).

The data of this clinical study were consistent with previous experimental studies, supporting reentry as the underlying mechanism of AF. All patients demonstrated non-uniform conduction around regions of bidirectional block resulting in multiple discrete wavefronts. Although anatomical obstacles such as the pulmonary and caval veins were involved in some reentrant circuits, reentry may also occur without the involvement of anatomical obstacles. Functional conduction block occurred throughout both atria and was sometimes associated with specific atrial structures such as the crista terminalis.

In Figure 1 four examples are shown of single isochronal maps as recorded during induced AF. In the upper left panel, a wavefront rotated

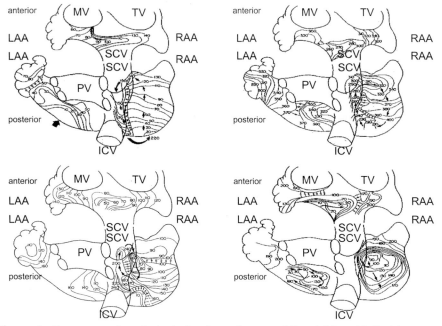

Figure 1. Four examples of single isochronal maps of the right and left atrium constructed during electrically induced AF in humans. The anterior and posterior surface of the atria are shown together in a 2-D plane. The maps were constructed using epicardial templates, containing 160 bipolar electrodes with an interelectrode distance ranging between 5 and 10 mm. The small arrows indicate the main direction of the activation waves. The thick arrow in the upper left panel points to retrograde activation from the ventricles at the site of the accessory pathway. SCV=superior caval vein, ICV=inferior caval vein, PV=pulmonary veins, RAA=right atrial appendage, LAA=left atrial appendage, MV=mitral valve, TV=tricuspid valve (modified from Cox et al.[8]).

counterclockwise around a line of conduction block along the sulcus terminalis. The upper right panel shows a large reentrant circuit propagating clockwise around a line of conduction block located both along the sulcus terminalis and in the free wall of the right atrium. In the lower left panel, the impulse propagated clockwise around a small area of conduction block located close to the superior caval vein. The lower right panel reveals a small reentrant circuit in the left atrium between the pulmonary veins and the mitral valve. In 6 of 13 patients, a reentrant circuit could be identified in the right atrium around the sulcus terminalis. In all patients, multiple wavefronts and lines of conduction block were found in both the right and left atrium. However, in the left atrium, reentrant circuits were more difficult to document and seemed to occur more fleetingly. A limitation of this first mapping study of human AF is that only *single* maps were presented and that beat-to-beat changes of the activation pattern during AF were not analysed.

High density mapping of electrically induced AF was performed by Konings et al. in 25 patients with the Wolff-Parkinson White syndrome.[9] During cardiac surgery, the free wall of the right and left atrium was mapped with a spoon electrode containing 244 unipolar electrodes (diameter 4 cm, spatial resolution 2.25 mm). The activation pattern of the right atrial free wall demonstrated a high intra- and inter-individual variation. The activation patterns ranged from well-organized activation consisting of a single planar wavefront to completely disorganized activation by multiple wavefronts propagating in different directions. The degree of organization was related to the frequency of AF, a long median cycle length being associated with a higher degree of organization and short median cycle lengths with more disorganized activation.

Based on the complexity of the activation, three different types of AF were distinguished. During type I AF, most of the time single broad wavefronts propagated across the right atrial free wall. Only small areas of slow conduction or conduction block occurred, not disturbing the main course of the large fibrillation waves. This type of AF probably reflects the presence of macro-reentry with involvement of anatomical obstacles.

During type II AF, either one wavefront propagating with marked local conduction delay or two separate wavefronts were present. During type III AF, in the mapping area with a diameter of 4 cm, multiple fibrillation waves were recorded being separated by functional lines of intraatrial conduction block. The incidence of type I, II, and III AF in this study population of 25 patients was 40%, 32%, and 28%, respectively.

In Figure 2, three specific phenomena (leading circle reentry, random reentry, focal activation) are shown, which could be observed in patients with type III AF. Isochronal maps of two consecutive beats of each phenomenon are shown together with a selection of unipolar electrograms. In the left panel, an example of leading circle is shown. The activation wave

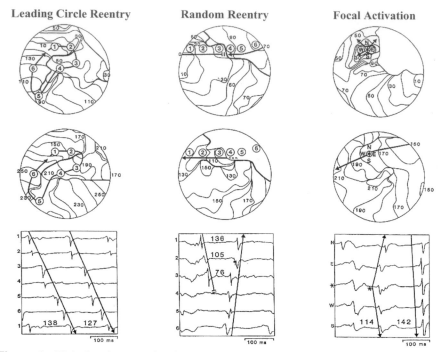

Figure 2. High density mapping (244 electrodes, diameter mapping area 3.6 cm) of the free wall of the right atrium during electrically induced type III AF in normal human atria. The maps show examples of leading circle reentry, random reentry and a focal activation pattern. Of each of these phenomena, two consecutive isochronal maps are given, together with a small selection of unipolar electrograms. See text for description (modified from Konings et al.[9]).

circulated clockwise around a shifting line of functional conduction block. These continuously shifting functional reentrant circuits were unstable and usually disappeared after a few beats. During random reentry, a wavefront re-excites an area that just has been activated by another fibrillation wave. In the middle panel, one wavefront activated the lower 2/3 of the mapping area from left to the right (t = 0−70 ms). The upper 1/3 of the mapping area was activated by another fibrillation wave from right to left, entering at t = 70 ms. The first wave activated electrodes 1 to 3 and was blocked between electrodes 3 and 4. The second wave activated electrodes 6 to 4 and was *not* blocked at electrode 3. Instead, it reentered the relative refractory tail of the first wave and re-excited electrodes 1, 2 and 3 in reverse order (second beat). The electrograms also show the first activation wavefront moving from electrode 1 to 3 and the second wavefront from electrode 6 to 1. Electrode 3 is reentered after only 76 ms showing that in humans the atrial refractory period during AF can be very short. In the right panels an example of focal activation is shown. During the first beat, a new wavefront arises in the upper part of the mapping area (*).

From here it spread radially into all directions. In the second beat, this focal activation pattern has disappeared again and the entire mapping area is now activated by a wavefront entering at the right and propagating to the left. During induced AF, such a focal activation pattern was only found as solitary events and never occurred repetitively. The electrogram recorded at the site of earliest activation (*) was preceded by a small r wave. This indicates that the focal activation pattern did not originate from a real focus, but rather is the result of epicardial breakthrough of an endocardial activation propagating through one of the pectinate muscles.

Chronic Atrial Fibrillation

So far, only four mapping studies have been performed in patients with chronic AF, mainly during cardiac surgery for mitral valve disease.[10-14] Holm et al.[10,11] analysed the activation patterns of the right atrial free wall and right atrial appendage in 16 patients. Using a mapping array of 56 bipolar electrodes, the occurrence of type I, II, and III patterns of AF was determined. At the posterior free wall, type I, II, and III AF was present in 27%, 40%, and 33% of the patients, respectively. In the right atrial appendage, the type of activation was 46% of type I, 27% of type II and 27% of type III. The major new finding of this study was that during *chronic* AF, focal activation in the right atrium occurred repetitively. The site of focal activation was consistently located at the right atrial appendage. An example is given in Figure 3. The left part shows the activation pattern of the right atrial appendage during 51 consecutive beats. The arrows indicate the main directions of activation. In the right part of the figure, the color maps of beats 33 to 43 are shown in more detail. During beat 33, two wavefronts entered the mapping area from different directions. In the next beat, the mapping area was again invaded by two wavefronts but simultaneously a third impulse arose in the center of the mapping area (*). During the next beats, this focal activation pattern repeated itself and during beats 33 to 43 the entire recording area was almost completely activated by a single radially spreading wavefront. During beat 44 this focal activation pattern disappeared and the mapping area was activated by multiple wavefronts.

Other mapping studies of chronic AF focussed on comparing right and left atrial activation which were mapped sequentially.[12,13] Surprisingly, in most patients, the activation of the left atrium was more organized. In 3 patients, organized and disorganized activation occurred alternately in the right atrium. However, since the mapping resolution of these studies was rather low, (only 30 unipolar or 24 bipolar electrodes) conduction abnormalities occurring in small areas could easily have been missed.

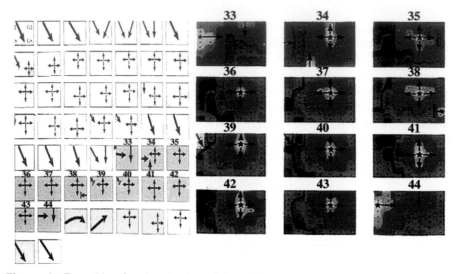

Figure 3. Repetitive focal activation of the right atrial appendage in a patient with chronic AF. In the left part, 51 consecutive activation maps are given diagrammatically. The right part shows a series of color maps elucidating a constant site of epicardial breakthrough. The activation maps were reconstructed with an epicardial template of 4 cm containing 56 bipolar electrodes with an interelectrode distance of 3 mm. The asterisks indicate the site of earliest activation (modified from Holm et al.[11]).

Noncontact mapping of the right atrium, both during induced (n=8) and chronic AF (n=3), could also distinguish three different types of AF.[14] In all patients, the right atrium was activated by wavefronts emerging from the septum either from the coronary sinus or Bachman's bundle. In this study, the majority of the patients showed a type III AF pattern.

Fibrillation Electrograms

The relation between the various morphologies of unipolar fibrillation electrograms and the spatial activation pattern during AF was first analysed by Konings et al.[15] Fibrillation electrograms were classified as singles, short doubles, long doubles and fragmented potentials. Long double potentials were specific for long lines of functional conduction block whereas fragmented potentials were observed both during pivoting of fibrillation waves and during slow conduction. In the normal human right atrium, no preferential sites for double potentials or fragmented electrograms were found.

The complexity of endocardial atrial activity during electrically induced AF was analysed by Jais et al. using a multipolar catheter (14 bipolar electrodes, 3 mm inter-electrode distance).[16] The study population consisted of 25 patients with paroxysmal AF. The complex electrical activity time was defined as the ratio of the total duration of electrograms with fibrillation intervals smaller than 100 ms and the total recording time. Atrial activity was more complex in the left than in the right atrium. In the right atrium, disorganized atrial activity at the postero-septal area abruptly changed to more organized activity in the anterior and lateral wall. This transition occurred at the crista terminalis. In the left atrium, atrial activity in the septum and the area between the pulmonary veins was more disorganized than in the appendage and the anterior left atrium. Thus, organized atrial activity appeared to be confined to the trabeculated parts of both the right and left atrium. The major limitation of this study was that only a small number of sites were analysed (four in the right and three in the left atrium).

Fragmentation Mapping

Kuck et al. used an electro-anatomical mapping system (CARTO) to analyse bipolar fibrillation electrograms in patients with paroxysmal AF.[17] Fibrillation electrograms were recorded during 45 seconds at multiple sites (36 ± 12) in the left atrium. Electrograms were classified as either type A (regular activation separated by a clear isoelectrical baseline), type B (irregular activation with perturbations of baseline and/or highly fragmented electrograms) or type C (alternation between type A and type B). Type B and C electrograms were equally present throughout the left atrium whereas the incidence of type A electrograms was higher in the upper left pulmonary vein.

In our institution, we are presently analysing the degree of fragmentation in unipolar electrograms recorded during mapping of the right and left atrium in patients with chronic AF undergoing cardiac surgery. In Figure 4 an example is given. The upper panel shows two successive beats during chronic AF in a patient with mitral valve disease. Multiple wavefronts enter the mapping area from different directions. The wavefronts are separated by lines of conduction block and frequently collide with each other. Sometimes, they can be seen pivoting around the end of a line of functional block. In the lower left panel, the different degree of fragmentation (singles, doubles, triples, quads, pentas, and continuous electrical activity) of fibrillation electrograms is illustrated. In the right lower panel a total fragmentation map is given representing the relative incidence of fragmented electrograms at each recording site. Fragmented electrograms were recorded at almost all electrodes. However, some sites showed a much higher incidence of fragmentation than others. It is yet unknown to what extent this spatial dispersion in fragmentation is due to the normal atrial architecture. It is a challenge for the future to elucidate whether fragmentation mapping of chronic AF can be used to diagnose the underlying electro-pathological substrate.

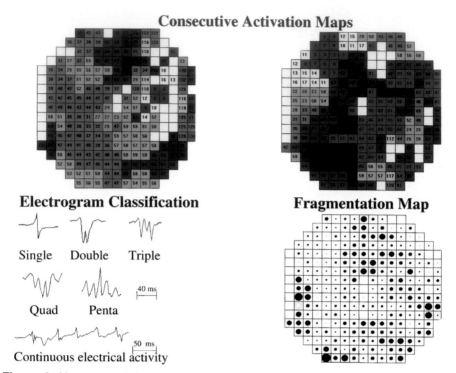

Figure 4. Upper panel: Activation maps of two successive beats during chronic AF recorded from the free wall of the right atrium in a patient with mitral valve disease. These maps were constructed using a spoon-shaped electrode (244 unipolar electrodes, 2.4 mm). Early activated areas are light colored and late activated areas are dark colored. Lower left panel: Classification of the degree of fragmentation of unipolar fibrillation electrograms. Lower right panel: Fragmentation map of the right atrial free wall during chronic AF. The size of each solid circle indicates the incidence of fragmentation.

References

1. Berbari EJ, Landr P, Geselowitz DB, et al. The methodology of cardiac mapping. In Shenasa M, Borggrefe M, Breithardt G (eds). **Cardiac Mapping**, Mount Kisco, New York, Futura Publishing;1993:11–34.
2. Jais P, Haissaguerre M, Shah DC, et al. A focal source of atrial fibrillation treated by discrete radiofrequency ablation. *Circulation* 1997;95:572–576.
3. Chen SA, Tai CT, Yu WC, et al. Right atrial focal atrial fibrillation: Electrophysiologic characteristics and radiofrequency catheter ablation. *J Cardiovasc Electrophysiol* 1999;10:328–335.
4. Melo J, Adragao PR, Neves J, et al. Electrosurgical treatment of atrial fibrillation with a new intraoperative radiofrequency ablation catheter. *Thorac Cardiovasc Surg* 1999;47 S3:370–372.
5. Haissaguerre M, Jais P, Gencel L, et al. Right and left atrial radiofrequency catheter therapy of paroxysmal atrial fibrillation. *J Cardiovasc Electrophysiol* 1996;7:1132–1144.

6. Kosakai Y, Kawaguchi AT, Isobe F, et al. Modified Maze procedure for patients with atrial fibrillation undergoing simultaneous open heart surgery. *Circulation* 1995;92:359–364.

7. Jessurun ER, Hemel van NM, Defauw JAMT, et al. Results of Maze surgery for lone paroxysmal atrial fibrillation. *Circulation* 2000;101:1559–1567.

8. Cox JL, Canavan TE, Schuessler RB, et al. The surgical treatment of atrial fibrillation. II. Intra-operative electrophysiologic mapping and description of the electrophysiologic basis of atrial flutter and atrial fibrillation. *J Thorac Cardiovasc Surg* 1991;101:406–426.

9. Konings KTS, Kirchhof CJ, Smeets JR, et al. High-density mapping of electrically induced atrial fibrillation in humans. *Circulation* 1994;89(4):1665–1680.

10. Holm M, Johansson R, Olsson SB, et al. A new method for analysis of atrial activation during chronic atrial fibrillation in man. *IEEE Transactions on Biomedical Engineering* 1996;43:198–210.

11. Holm M, Johansson R, Brandt J, et al. Epicardial right atrial free wall mapping in chronic atrial fibrillation. Documentation of repetitive activation with a focal spread—a hitherto unrecognised phenomenon in man. *Eur Heart J* 1997 18(2):290–310.

12. Harada A, Sasaki K, Fukushima T, et al. Atrial activation during chronic atrial fibrillation in patients with isolated mitral valve disease. *Ann Thorac Surg* 1996;61:104–112.

13. Sueda T, Nagata H, Shikata H, et al. Simple left atrial procedure for chronic atrial fibrillation associated with mitral valve disease. *Ann Thorac Surg* 1996;62(6):1796–1800.

14. Schilling RJ, Kadish AH, Peters NS, et al. Endocardial mapping of atrial fibrillation in the human right atrium using a non-contact catheter. *Eur Heart J* 2000;21(7):550–564.

15. Konings KTS, Smeets JRLM, Penn OC, et al. Configuration of unipolar atrial electrograms during electrically induced atrial fibrillation. *Circulation* 1997;95:1231–1241.

16. Jais P, Haissaguerre M, Shah DC, et al. Regional disparities of endocardial atrial activation in paroxysmal atrial fibrillation. *Pacing Clin Electrophysiol* 1996;19:1998–2003.

17. Kuck KH, Ernst S, Cappato R, et al. Nonfluoroscopic endocardial catheter mapping of atrial fibrillation. *J Cardiovasc Electrophysiol* 1998;9:S57–S62.

Chapter 2

The Role of Deteriorated Inferoposterior Interatrial Conduction in Atrial Fibrillation

S. Bertil Olsson, MD, PhD

Introduction

Over the last years, great interest has been paid to the mechanism whereby atrial fibrillation (AF) starts. One important observation has been that many patients with paroxysmal AF have abundant ectopic atrial beats, originating in the pulmonary venous muscular shaft and even sometimes in the atrial wall or the proximal part of the superior caval vein. Less interest has been paid to the initial substrate, where the excitation wave deteriorates into a more complex pattern, ultimately resulting in AF. As summarized in this chapter, there is growing evidence that deterioration of inter-atrial conduction plays an important role at this phase of the initiation of AF.

Anatomic Evidence

Human atria are developed with a double-layer septal structure, resulting in not only a separation of the atrial cavities but also a separation of the muscle structures of the right and left atrium. There are, however, both macro- and microscopic muscular structures connecting the atria, constituting the prerequisite for transseptal conduction of the excitation wave.

The macroscopic muscular connections between the atria have long been identified.[1] Figure 1 left illustrates the gross muscular connection be-

From Virag N, Blanc O, Kappenberger L (eds): *Computer Simulation and Experimental Assessment of Cardiac Electrophysiology.* ©Futura Publishing Co., Inc., Armonk, NY, 2001.

tween the anterior parts of right and left atrium respectively, depicted in 1835. This connection, after having been rediscovered almost 100 years later and named the Bachmann bundle, is however not a constant macro-anatomical finding.[2] In addition to the Bachmann bundle, there are often one or more anterior interatrial muscle bridges in the same area.[3]

Other macroscopic inter-atrial myocardial connections are found at the inferoposterior portion of the interatrial space (see Figure 1 right). These bundles are often multiple and extend from below or above the pulmonary veins[3] towards the adjacent right atrial myocardium. Others cannot verify a wide distribution of these connections but instead find them inserting in close proximity although not immediately adjacent to the coronary sinus ostium (Platonov, unpublished observations). Cardiac muscular bundles of proarrhythmic importance are usually identified as eponyms. Since Bourgery was the first to illustrate the position of the inferoposterior interatrial bundles, and Platonov the first to document the importance of deteriorated conduction along their route, it is pertinent to hereafter name these as the Bourgery-Platonov bundles.

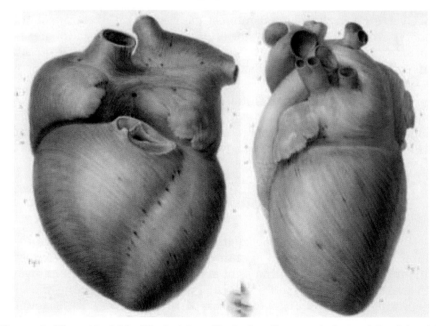

Figure 1. The oldest identified picture illustrating the morphology of the interatrial muscular connections. The left figure illustrates the anterior interatrial connection, later named the Bachmann bundle. Note that the fibers of this muscle bundle connect to the different atrial at a distance from the septal structure shared by both atria but also that the figure suggests a muscular continuity across these septal raphae. The right figure depicts the inferoposterior muscular connections, inserting in the right atrial septal wall close to the ostium of the coronary sinus. Lithographs after original drawing by NH Jacob, published by JM Bourgery.[1]

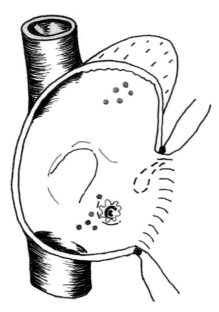

Figure 2. Schematic illustration of localization of right atrial insertions of macro- or microscopical muscular inter-atrial connections, indicated by green color. Note that the insertions of both the Bachmann and the Bourgery-Platonov bundles may be multiple. For further information, see text.

The microscope reveals additional muscular interatrial connections. Thus, the wall of the coronary sinus holds myocardial fibers, connecting at its orifice with the right atrial myocardium and also to the left atrial wall via tiny connections.[4] In addition, there is a microscopic muscular continuity along the raphae of the septal isthmus, projected on the septal right atrial surface around the fossa ovalis. It is unclear whether this muscular continuity is patchy or can be followed all around the true septum.

The muscular connections between the right and the left atrium are thus multiple, often tiny, spatially well separated and are subject to great interindividual variability (Figure 2). It should also be underlined that the exact transitions from the muscular interatrial connections to the proper atrial myocardium are still poorly studied. However, the delicate anatomy of these routes offers an obvious prerequisite for structural damages with a probable impact on the interatrial conduction.

The Normal Interatrial Conduction

Using epicardial mapping technique on the surgically exposed human heart, the left atrial activation during sinus rhythm appears at two distinctly separated areas.[5] Depending upon the localization of the exit of the sinus node, the initial activation at these different areas may differ temporally. During sinus rhythm, initial left atrial activation is however identified anteriorly and inferoposteriorly, coinciding with the insertions of the Bachmann and Bourgery-Platonov bundles, respectively. After spreading along the left atrium, the excitation wavefronts collide at the posterior surface of the left atrium, between the pulmonary veins.

Electroanatomical endocardial excitation analysis of the left atrium during sinus rhythm reveals two areas of early excitation, again in agreement with the left atrial insertion of the macroscopic interatrial bundles.[6]

The impulse conduction from the left to the right atrium follows the same routes. The earliest sign of right atrial endocardial activation at left atrial stimulation varies with the site of stimulation in patients who normally have sinus rhythm.[7] Thus, left atrial pacing from the distal coronary sinus is followed by early activation at the posterior part of the right interatrial septum. The exact place is mostly in close vicinity of the ostium of the coronary sinus, i.e. at the right atrial insertion of the Bourgery-Platonov bundles or at the septal insertion of the fibers running in the wall of the coronary sinus. When the pacing is performed from a more anterior location in the left atrium, early right atrial activation can be found at the site of the insertion of the Bachmann bundle.

Deterioration of Anterior Interatrial Conduction

Advanced interatrial block is associated with atypical atrial flutter[8] is evidenced by a specific morphology of the P wave, compatible with a conduction block in the Bachmann bundle.[9] When these patients are in sinus rhythm, the gross activation of the left atrium has the opposite direction as that of the right atrium, implying that the right-to-left activation must take place inferoposteriorly, i.e., at the site of the Bourgery-Platonov bundles. The interpretation of the pathoelectrophysiological reason for the abnormal P wave morphology at advanced interatrial block is further supported by the fact that surgical interruption of the Bachmann bundle makes the P wave change into a similar morphology as recorded in these patients.[10]

Deterioration of Inferoposterior Interatrial Conduction

Based upon the assumption that deterioration of interatrial conduction also may occur in the inferoposterior interatrial connections, we explored the activation sequence of the atria by signal-averaged P wave recording and orthogonal vector lead technique.[11] The terminal phase of the P wave, and its spatial direction differed significantly between a group of patients with paroxysmal AF without significant prolongation of the P wave and an age-matched control group. The direction of the later part of the P vector was thus compatible with a collision of the left atrial excitation waves closer to the interatrial septum in the AF patients in comparison with the control group. This finding therefore suggests that the right-to-left inferoposterior conduction is significantly impaired in this group of patients.

Using multiple multipolar electrode catheter technique for intracardiac excitation analysis in another group of patients with paroxysmal AF, Platonov et al. localized the interatrial conduction delay to the vicinity of the ostium of the coronary sinus.[12] Conduction times between distal coronary sinus, posterior right atrial septum and lateral right atrium, measured during regular pacing at these respective locations, did thus differ between the patient group and a control group in a similar way, irrespective of the pacing position, suggesting the conduction delay to take place within the posterior part of the septum within the right atrium. In contrast, the marked exaggeration of conduction delay, which occurred during early ectopic beats, initiated from the distal coronary sinus, was localized to the proximal part of the coronary sinus, within 10 mm from its ostium. Taken together, the verified pathoelectrophysiologic properties of inferoposterior interatrial connections and right atrial septal wall constitute a possible initial substrate where impulse conduction may deteriorate into a more complex pattern. Indeed, the majority of spontaneously occurring attacks of AF in those patients seemed to originate from this area.[13]

Although the myocardial continuity across the raphae of the interatrial septum may be a further prerequisite for transseptal impulse conduction, convincing evidence is still lacking that human interatrial conduction utilizes these fibers.

How can the Findings be Interpreted?

Among the different pathoelectrophysiological findings observed in patients with AF, deterioration of the inferoposterior interatrial conduction can be added to several earlier well documented findings. The abundance of the present finding in several separate patient groups, using different investigation techniques, suggests that it may be a prerequisite for the arrhythmia in a large number of patients. Whether the finding is a primary pathoelectrophysiological defect or a consequence of a structural and/or electrical remodeling caused by AF is still an open question.

Obviously, we are still lacking the complete knowledge of how different interatrial myocardial structures participate in the transseptal conduction in individuals with normal sinus rhythm as well as in patients with AF and other atrial arrhythmias. Today's knowledge can, however, be summarized in the highly simplified electroanatomical cartoon of the atria, the interatrial structures and their possible proarrhythmic role as in Figure 3.

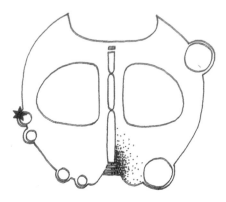

Figure 3. Cartoon of the atrial myocardium with special reference to the possible role of interatrial conduction in atrial fibrillation. The star indicates a likely origin of an ectopic impulse while the dotted surface corresponds to the area of the suggested initial substrate where the conducted impulse deteriorates into atrial fibrillation.

In summary, the current observations suggest an appealing localized pro-arrhythmic mechanism, theoretically possible to counteract in several different ways, i.e., by electrical insulation or elimination, using anatomically or electrophysiologically guided ablation and pacing techniques.

References

1. Bourgery JM. Traité complet de l'anatomie de l'homme. Paris 1831–1854.
2. Mikhailov S and Chukbar A. Topographic anatomy of the cardiac conductive system (in Russian language). *Atat Arch* 1982;6:56–66.
3. Ho SY, Sanchez-Quintana D, Cabrera JA, et al. Anatomy of the left atrium: Implications for radiofrequency ablation of atrial fibrillation. *J Cardiovasc Electrophysiol* 1999;10:1525–1533.
4. Chauvin M, Shah D, Haïssaguerre M, et al. The anatomic basis of connections between the coronary sinus musculature and the left atrium in humans. *Circulation* 2000;101:647–652.
5. Boineau JP, Canavan TE, Schuessler RB, et al. Demonstration of a widely distributed atrial pacemaker complex in the human heart. *Circulation* 1988; 77:1221–1223.
6. Shah D, Haïssaguerre M, Jais P, et al. Dual input right to left atrial activation correlating with P wave morphology. *Pacing Clinical Electrophysiol* 1999; 22:832.
7. Roithinger FX, Cheng JC, SippensGroenewegen A, et al. Use of electroanatomic mapping to delineate transseptal atrial conduction in humans. *Circulation* 1999;100:1791–1797.
8. Daubert C, Gras D, Berder V, et al. Permanent atrial resynchronization by synchronous biatrial pacing in the preventive treatment of atrial flutter associated with high degree interatrial block. *Arch Mal Coeur Vaiss* 1994;87(suppl 11):1535–1546.
9. Bayés de Luna A, Cladellas M, Otter R, et al. Interatrial conduction block and retrograde activation of the left atrium and paroxysmal supraventricular tachyarrhythmia. *Eur Heart J* 1988;9:1112–1118.

10. Waldo AL, Bush HL, Gelband H, et al. Effects on the canine P wave of discrete lesions in the specialized atrial tracts. *Circ Res* 1971;29:452–461.
11. Platonov PG, Carlson J, Ingemansson MP, et al. Detection of inter-atrial conduction defects with unfiltered signal-averaged P-wave ECG in patients with lone atrial fibrillation. *Europace* 2000;2:32–41.
12. Platonov PG, Yuan S, Hertervig E, et al. Further evidence of localised posterior interatrial conduction delay in lone paroxysmal atrial fibrillation. *Europace* 2001 (in press).
13. Platonov PG, Yuan S, Hertervig E, et al. Localisation of the initial fibrillatory cycle in patients with paroxysmal atrial fibrillation. *Scandinavian CV J* 2001 (in press).

Chapter 3

Simulation of Arrhythmias in a Computer Model of Human Atria

Olivier Blanc, MS, Nathalie Virag, PhD,
Andre Nicoulin, PhD, Vincent Jacquemet, MS,
Jean-Marc Vesin, PhD, Lukas Kappenberger, MD

Introduction

Computer modeling of the heart could significantly improve our understanding of what occurs during cardiac arrhythmias by allowing simulation of experiments that cannot be done *in vivo*. The success of such an approach, however, depends on how the computer model can represent a correct approximation of actual electrophysiological behavior.[1]

Atrial arrhythmias are the most frequent arrhythmias in humans. Today, most of the treatments for atrial fibrillation (AF) are based on empirical considerations and many underlying mechanisms remain unclear. Developing a computer model of atria requires consideration of both physiological and anatomic details. However, since available computation time is limited, each model requires a compromise between the following parameters: complexity of the membrane model, complexity of tissue structure (monodomain/bidomain),[1] size of tissue and number of spatial nodes, complexity of the represented anatomy, duration of the simulated events, and stability and accuracy of the numerical method.

In contrast to the ventricular myocardium, the limited surface and wall thickness of the atria should allow the development of a realistic

[1] This study was made possible by grants from the Theo-Rossi-Di-Montelera Foundation, Medtronic Europe and the Swiss Governmental Commission of Innovative Technologies (CTI).

From Virag N, Blanc O, Kappenberger L (eds): *Computer Simulation and Experimental Assessment of Cardiac Electrophysiology.* ©Futura Publishing Co., Inc., Armonk, NY, 2001.

model with today's computer power. Such computer models of atria taking into account anatomy have been recently proposed.[2,3] Our objective is to construct a model delivering simulation results that could reproduce clinical arrhythmias. This means that our computer model, based on membrane ionic kinetics, will have to be able to simulate atrial arrhythmias during several seconds in a tissue with realistic size. To achieve this goal, we selected a simplified cellular model (Beeler-Reuter[4] model) and tissue structure (monodomain[1] model), and then implemented a three-dimensional simplified anatomy with only one layer of cells and introduced only the main anatomic features (the veins and the valves).

Description of the Computer Model

Based on the assumption that atria are constituted of thin walls, we built our anatomic model of the right and left atria by folding a two-dimensional cardiac tissue into a model with a three-dimensional structure of one layer of cells. This simplified structure is composed of two connected ellipsoids with a diameter of 35 mm and a total length of 80 mm. Orifices of appropriate size and location have been placed to simulate the veins and the valves (Figure 1). The surface of the mitral valve and the tricuspid valve is 4 cm^2, 2 cm^2 for the superior vena cava, 2.5 cm^2 for the inferior vena cava and 1 cm^2 for each pulmonary vein. No conduction is assumed through the septum, and other local tissue characteristics, such

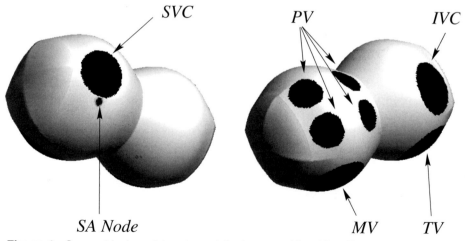

Figure 1. Geometrical model proposed for human atria with orifices represented in black. On the left is an anterior view with the right atrium on the left, and on the right is the posterior view with the right atrium on the right.

as fiber orientation or pectinate muscles, have not been taken into account. The tissue is homogeneous and isotropic. Therefore, this simplified model takes into account only the effect of the large anatomical obstacles created by the veins and valves in a model with a realistic size.

For the cardiac tissue, we have implemented a monodomain model and the ionic kinetics is given by the well-known Beeler-Reuter model.[4] This model has been developed for the ventricles, but as a first approximation, we use it for an atrial tissue. The use of an atrial cellular model[5] would increase significantly computation time and we made the assumption that the general behavior would be very similar. Moreover, the use of a bidomain model would imply a slowing of the computation speed by at least one order of magnitude.

The propagation equation is solved using firstly an explicit computation of the membrane ionic current and secondly a semi-implicit current diffusion.[6] The choice of the time and space discretization is the result of a tradeoff between computation speed and accuracy. Computer simulations of electrical propagation and especially reentry simulations impose strong requirements on spatial discretization.[7] Based on numerical simulations with different space steps, we choose a spatial discretization of 200 μm, corresponding to a total of about 250,000 nodes. The time discretization is 25 μs. This model has been implemented with double precision on standard PCs. For 250,000 nodes, the computation time on one processor of a Pentium III 500 MHz takes 16 hours per second of simulated time, and the RAM occupied by the model is 250 MB.

Atrial Arrhythmias

The propagation of a normal sinus beat is initiated by injecting an intracellular current into the cells of the sinoatrial node region (SA node), defined anatomically at the superior vena cava right atrial junction. Atrial arrhythmias can be initiated using a programmed stimulation protocol similar to that used for electrophysiological studies.

Atrial flutter-like activity was initiated, displaying as a single macroreentrant circuit with a periodic pattern. Atrial fibrillation was initiated with a normal sinus rhythm followed by two or three *critically timed and located ectopic beats*, with an overall propagation velocity decreased from 90 cm/s to 30 cm/s. We have been able to initiate AF sustained for more than 40 seconds (corresponding to about 25 days of computation time). Interestingly, however, most AF spontaneously converted to atrial flutter or sinus rhythm, as in biological models. Figure 2 illustrates an example of initiating AF by two ectopic beats located in the high right atrium with coupling intervals of 320 ms and 222 ms, respectively. In this case, after an initiation phase, fibrillation lasts for about 8 seconds

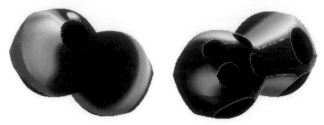

t = 590 ms

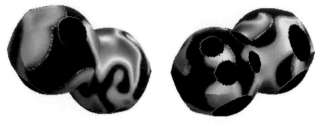

t = 4400 ms

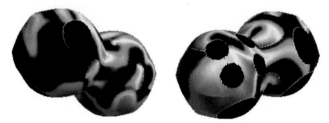

t = 9600 ms

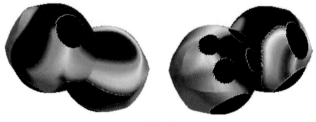

t = 13700 ms

-80 mV   20 mV

Figure 2. Example of initiation of atrial fibrillation in a homogeneous tissue with a propagation velocity of 30 cm/s and APD = 252 ms. The sinus rhythm is followed by two ectopic beats with a coupling interval of 350 ms and 222 ms, respectively. Top image: shortly after the application of the second ectopic beat, creation of a reentrant wavefront. Two middle images: during atrial fibrillation with up to eight independent wavelets. Bottom image: atrial flutter-like activity with a periodic pattern.

and then finally converts to sustained atrial flutter. Similarly to what has been mapped in humans, AF displays as multiple reentering wavelets (four to eight) traveling randomly.[8,9]

The Effect of Anatomy

One important observation is that in our model atrial arrhythmias are a combination of functional and anatomical reentries and therefore that the geometry plays an important role. Indeed, the effect of heart anatomy on the mechanisms of arrhythmia is clearly visible in our experiments. The orifices simulating the veins and arteries create wavefront propagation pathways or preferential regions for wavefront collision. On one hand, anatomical obstacles tend to break wavefronts, and we have identified that the isthmus between inferior vena cava and tricuspid valve and the pulmonary veins region are critical for the initiation of arrhythmias. On the other hand, anatomical obstacles act like anchors for the reentrant wave and have a stabilization effect.[10] Indeed, during the initiation of AF by two ectopic beats, a rotor is created that rotated around the superior vena cava. After several rotations, the wave is detached and hits a slow recovery wave front, initiating the AF. The transition from fibrillation to a periodic and more stable reentrant wave is facilitated due to the anchoring phenomenon. It seems that the vena cava play an important role in the anchoring process.

We also measured histogram of activation intervals during AF, as represented in Figure 3. Figure 4 shows how these fibrillation activation intervals are spatially distributed on the atrial surface: we observe a higher rate in the left atrium than in the right. This shows that, even in a homogeneous tissue, anatomical obstacles can create a non-uniform spatial distribution of rate. Therefore, these obstacles are important in determining the size and location of reentrant pathways, which will in turn determine the rate.

It is interesting to observe what happens when the anatomical obstacles are removed from the tissue while AF is running, as represented in Figure 5. We can observe that the spatial distribution of AF activation intervals becomes much more uniform (the differences between right and left atrium disappears) and that the overall rate is higher.

Conclusion

We proposed here a simplified model of human atria. It has the advantage of having a low computational load, which has been obtained by making some important simplifications: modeling of only one layer of

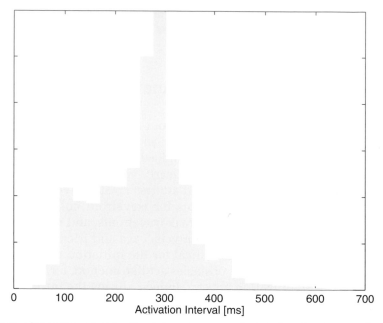

Figure 3. Histogram of activation intervals, computed during the 8 seconds of sustained AF presented in Figure 2. The mean activation interval is 253 ms, corresponding to a rate of 237 bpm.

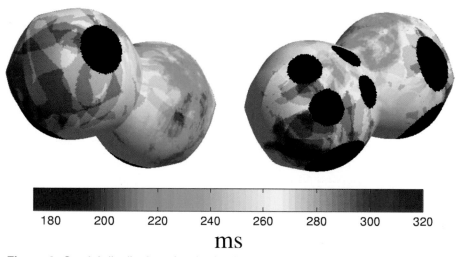

Figure 4. Spatial distribution of activation intervals during atrial fibrillation. For each point on the atrial surface, a mean activation interval was computed over the 8 seconds of sustained AF presented in Figure 2.

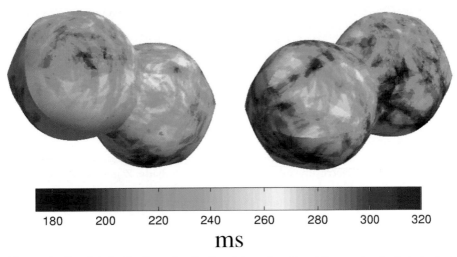

180   200   220   240   260   280   300   320
ms

Figure 5. Spatial distribution of activation intervals without the anatomical obstacles. For each point on the atrial surface, a mean activation interval was computed over 7 seconds, starting one second after the anatomical obstacles have been removed.

cells, simplified geometry, use of Beeler-Reuter model and uniform properties for the whole atrial tissue. However, it can reproduce atrial arrhythmias having a size of reentrant circuit, a rate and a number of wavelets similar to what has been observed in biological experiments.

This simple model allowed us to study the importance of large anatomical obstacles on AF. Indeed, atrial geometry is one factor that is known to have an influence on atrial arrhythmias.[11] In addition to anatomical obstacles, other anatomical factors, such as atrial anisotropy and heterogeneities, or functional factors, such as nonuniform repolarization, could be also studied with minor changes in this computer model. The advantage of computer simulations in this case, is that it is possible to study *separately*, in controlled and reproducible conditions, the effect of these factors. Finally, in a next step this model will be used to study therapeutic interventions for AF (see Chapter 16).

References

1. Henriquez CS, Papazoglou AA. Using computer models to understand the roles of tissue structure and membrane dynamics in arrhythmogenesis. *Proc of the IEEE* 1996;84:334–354.
2. Gray RA, Jalife J. Ventricular fibrillation and atrial fibrillation are two different beasts. *Chaos* 1998;8:65–78.
3. Harrild DM, Henriquez CS. A computer model of normal conduction in the human atria. *Circ Res* 2000;87:e25–e36.

4. Beeler GW, Reuter H. Reconstruction of the action potential of ventricular myocardial fibers. *J Physiol* 1977;268:177–210.
5. Nygren A, Fiset C, Clark JW, et al. Mathematical model of an adult human atrial cell: The role of K+ currents in repolarization. *Circ Res* 1998;82:63–81.
6. Virag N, Vesin J-M, Kappenberger L. A computer model of cardiac electrical activity for the simulation of arrhythmias. *Pacing Clinical Electrophysiol* 1998;21(Part II): 2366–2371.
7. Wu J, Zipes DP. Effects of spatial segmentation in the continuous model of excitation propagation in cardiac muscle. *J Cardiovasc Electrophysiol* 1999; 10:965–972.
8. Allessie MA, Rensma PL, Brugada J, et al. Pathophysiology of Atrial Fibrillation. **Cardiac Electrophysiology From Cell to Bedside**, Zipes DP, Jalife J (eds), WB Saunders, Philadelphia 1990: 48–559.
9. Schilling RJ, Kadish AH, Peters NS, et al. Endocardial mapping of atrial fibrillation in the human right atrium using a non-contact catheter. *Eur Heart J* 2000;21:550–564.
10. Xie F, Qu Z, Garfinkel A. Dynamics of reentry around a circular obstacle in cardiac tissue. *Physical Review E* 1998;58:6355–6358.
11. Cox JL, Schuessler RB, Boineau JP. The surgical treatment of atrial fibrillation: I. Summary of the current concepts of the mechanisms of atrial flutter and atrial fibrillation. *J Thorac Cardiovasc Surg* 1991;101:402–405.

Chapter 4

A Realistic and Efficient Model of Excitation Propagation in the Human Atria

Christian W. Zemlin, MS, Hanspeter Herzel, PhD,
Siew Y. Ho, PhD, FRCPath, Alexandre Panfilov, PhD

Introduction

Atrial arrhythmias are clinically important because they are so common. Atrial fibrillation (AF) alone occurs in 0.4% to 0.9% of the general population and in 2% to 4% of people above 60 years.[1,2] As longevity increases, so does the need to develop therapies for AF.

To understand the mechanisms underlying atrial arrhythmias, various approaches are needed, from clinical studies and electrophysiological experiments to theoretical modeling of wave propagation in atrial tissue. In this chapter, we discuss the feasibility of a realistic model of anatomy and electrical activity of the atria. Starting with Moe[3], there have been a number of atrial models.[4–7] These models deliberately use a simplified geometry and models of electrical activity that differ considerably from that of human atrial cells. Recently, an anatomically accurate three-dimensional model of the atria was developed by Harrild and Henriquez.[8] They used a three-dimensional finite volume method and the Lindblad model[9] of atrial electrical activity. The Harrild/Henriquez model was able to describe accurately the normal atrial activation sequence. However, since iterative integration methods in three-dimensions are used, extensive computations are necessary and it is difficult to study reentrant arrhythmias using this model. Furthermore, the model does not incorporate anisotropy of the atrial walls, which is known to be pronounced.

From Virag N, Blanc O, Kappenberger L (eds): *Computer Simulation and Experimental Assessment of Cardiac Electrophysiology.* ©Futura Publishing Co., Inc., Armonk, NY, 2001.

Our goal is to develop an anatomically accurate and numerically efficient model that makes modeling reentrant arrhythmias feasible at low computational cost. The emphasis of this chapter is on the construction of the model rather than the preliminary results.

Model Construction and Results

Anatomically, the human atria have quite a complex three-dimensional geometry. However, as we are interested in wave propagation only, we can consider the atrial walls and the septum as two-dimensional. This means that we assume excitation occurs only along and not transversely across the thin walls. In this way, we can drastically simplify boundary conditions and reduce the computational cost. The muscular bundles that are preferential conduction pathways (crista terminalis, pectinate muscles, Bachmann's bundle) will be treated as quasi-one-dimensional structures.

Our primary source for anatomical atrial data is the Visible Human Project (http://www.nlm.gov/pubs/visible_human.html). It provides voxel data of two human bodies. Freudenberg et al. segmented these data[10] and provided us with a data set describing the human atria (see Figure 1). From the voxel data we generated a triangular surface representing human atria using the Marching Cubes isosurfacing algorithm[11] generalized[12] which allows to find not only the outer surface of the atria but the septal surface as well. The resulting triangulated isosurface is shown in Figure 2. It consists of roughly 66,000 triangles. For proper description of wave propagation we have further subdivided each triangle into 9 triangles and obtained a surface composed of approximately 600,000 triangles with an average side length of 0.28 mm.

The atria are strongly anisotropic. The conduction speed along the long axis of the myocyte fiber is about three times that in the direction orthogonal to the fibers.[13] The information regarding typical orientations of gross fibers was obtained from dissections of anatomical specimens. We copied these fiber orientations manually onto views from different angles of our model and projected them onto the underlying triangles. We used interpolation for the triangles that did not receive a fiber orientation this way. We also include pectinate muscles and the crista terminalis. They are important for the activation sequence, because conduction velocity in these bundles is still higher than the velocity in fiber direction in the remaining atrial surface.[13] In our model, the pectinate muscles are modeled as triangle strips that are connected to the atrial surface (see Figure 3). This way, they behave as one-dimensional cables, and we have a uniform description of all parts of our model.

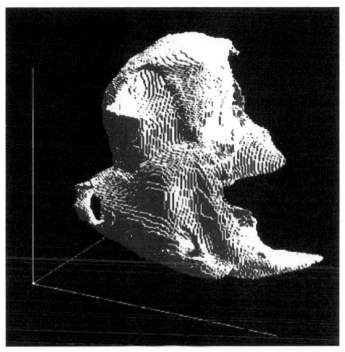

Figure 1. Voxel representation of the atria as provided from the Visible Human Project.

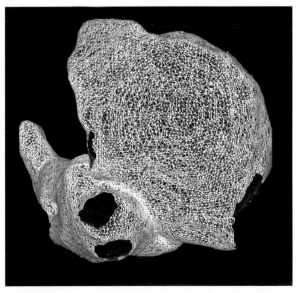

Figure 2. Triangular mesh gained using the Generalized Marching Cubes Algorithm. See text for details.

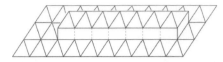

Figure 3. Modeling of crista terminalis and pectinate muscles. These special conduction pathways are modeled as triangle strips that are connected to the atrial wall at their beginning, their end, and to a lesser degree in between.

A crucial step in the construction of a realistic and efficient model is the choice of a model for electrical activity of the atrial cells. We try to get the predictive power of the most detailed ionic models[9,14] at reduced computational cost. Starting from the Courtemanche et al. model,[14] we reduced the number of variables from 19 to 6. We made sure that the reduced model well retains the restitution and dispersion properties of the original model as well as its action potential shape and the dependency of action potential shape on stimulation frequency. The reduction resulted in a speed gain of about a factor of 5.

Having thus defined the geometry and the dynamics of electrical activity, we need to solve the equations:

$$\frac{\partial V}{\partial t}(x,t) = f(V,s) + \nabla \cdot (DV)$$

$$\frac{\partial s}{\partial t}(x,t) = g(V,s) \tag{1}$$

where V is the transmembrane potential, s is the vector of gating variables of the simplified model, D is the diffusion tensor (reflecting the fiber orientation of the atria). The functions f and g specify our tissue model. The reaction terms of Equation 1 are integrated using a standard Rush-Larsen algorithm.[15] To approximate the diffusion term in Equation 1, we rely on Gauss' theorem. Consider the neighborhood of some vertex p of interest (Figure 4). We assume that ∇V is linear on each of the triangles

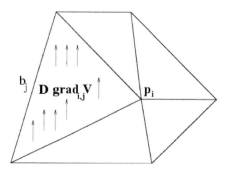

Figure 4. Illustration of Gauss' Method to estimate diffusion. See text for details.

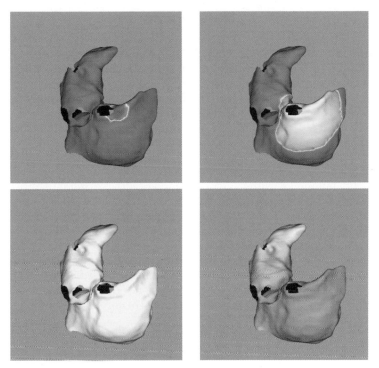

Figure 5. The sinus rhythm in our atrial model. The view is from above, the hole next to the red spot in the first picture is the superior vena cava. Color encodes trans-membrane voltage, blue meaning resting potential and red maximal depolarization. Snapshots are taken after 0 ms, 30 ms, 100 ms, and 220 ms.

adjacent to p. This allows us to calculate the flow $D\nabla V$ on each of these triangles, and dividing by their total area, we get an approximation of $\nabla (D\nabla V)$ (according to Gauss' law).

Here we show only preliminary results to demonstrate the feasibility of our approach. Figure 5 shows a series of snapshots from the simulation of a sinus rhythm in our model. The computation time needed for 220 ms real time is 150 minutes on a Pentium III/600.

Our development of a realistic atrial model is just at the beginning. We have shown that using our approach we can construct the anatomical atrial model and effectively study wave propagation in it. Further work needs to be done on tuning our model and comparison of our computational results with the results of experimental studies of wave propagation in atria.

We thank Jan Freudenberg for providing us with voxel data of the atria and Johannes Schmidt-Ehrenberg for help with the Generalized Marching Cubes Algorithm.

References

1. Kannel WB, Abbott RD, Savage DD, et al. Epicemiologic features of chronic atrial fibrillation: The Framingham study. *N Engl J Med* 1982;306(17): 1018–1022.
2. Camm AJ. **Nonpharmocological Treatment of Atrial Fibrillation**, Preface. Armonk, New York. Futura Publishing Company, 1997.
3. Moe G, Reinbold W, Abildskov J. A computer model of atrial fibrillation. *Am Heart J* 1964;67:200–220.
4. Macchi E. Digital-computer simulation of the atrial electrical excitation cycle in man. *Adv Cardiol* 1974;10:102–110.
5. Kafer CJ. Internodal pathways in the human atria: A model study. *Comput Biomed Res* 1991;24:549–563.
6. Lorange M, Gulrajani RM. A computer heart model incorporating anisotropic propagation, I: Model construction and simulation of normal activation. *J Electrocardiol* 1993;26:245–260.
7. Killmann R, Wach P, Dienstl F. Three-dimensional computer model of the entire human heart for simulation of reentry and tachycardia: Gap phenomenon and Wolff-Parkinson-White syndrome. *Basic Res Cardiol* 1991;86:485–501.
8. Harrild DM, Henriquez CS. A computer model of normal conduction in the human atria. *Circ Res* 2000;87:e25–e36.
9. Nygren A, Fiset C, Firek L, et al. Mathematical model of an adult human atrial cell. *Circ Res* 1998;82:63–81.
10. Freudenberg J, Schiemann T, Tiede U, et al. Simulation of cardiac excitation patterns in a three-dimensional anotomical heart atlas. *Computers in Biology and Medicine* 2000;30:191–203.
11. Lorensen WE, Cline HE. Marching cubes: A high resolution 3D construction algorithm. *Computer Graphics* 1987 (Proceedings of SIGGRAPH '87);21(4): 163–169.
12. Hege H, Seebaβ M, Stalling D, et al. A generalized marching cubes algorithm based on non-binary classifications. *ZIB Preprint* 1997;SC:97–105.
13. Saffitz JE, Yamada KJ. Gap junction distribution in the heart. In: **Cardiac Electrophysiology**. Philadelphia, WB Saunders, 2000:179–187.
14. Courtemanche M, Ramirez RJ, Nattel S. Ionic mechanisms underlying human atrial action potential properties: Insights from a mathematical model. *Amer J Physiol* 1998;275:H301–H321.
15. Rush S, Larsen H. A practical algorithm for solving dynamic membrane equations. *IEEE Trans on BME* 1978;25:389–392.

Part II.

Electrical Mapping and Modeling of Ventricles

Chapter 5

Noninvasive Electrocardiographic Imaging of Cardiac Excitation and Arrhythmia

Yoram Rudy, PhD

Introduction

The development of a reliable noninvasive imaging modality for cardiac electrical function has been an important goal of electrocardiographic research. Given the rapid increase in our understanding of the mechanisms of cardiac arrhythmias and the growing arsenal of (invasive and noninvasive) interventions, such a modality is needed for specific diagnosis, localization, and guided therapy. In previous studies,[1,2] we validated and demonstrated that a noninvasive electrocardiographic imaging (ECGI) method developed in our laboratory[3] can reconstruct epicardial potentials, electrograms and isochrones from measured body surface potentials with good accuracy. In particular, single and multiple foci of arrhythmic activity (simulated by myocardial pacing) were localized with better than 10 mm accuracy, and electrograms and isochrones during such activity were faithfully reconstructed. A major step towards the clinical application of ECGI is its evaluation in abnormal hearts in the presence of structural heart disease, and during reentrant arrhythmias in the abnormal electrophysiological substrates of such hearts. This chapter summarizes two recent studies in infarcted hearts, in which the ability of ECGI to detect and characterize abnormal electrophysiological (EP) substrates and to image reentrant arrhythmias was demonstrated. These studies were conducted in collaboration with Bruno Taccardi's laboratory at the University of Utah and described in detail in recent publications.[4,5]

From Virag N, Blanc O, Kappenberger L (eds): *Computer Simulation and Experimental Assessment of Cardiac Electrophysiology.* ©Futura Publishing Co., Inc., Armonk, NY, 2001.

Imaging Electrophysiologically Abnormal Substrates: Myocardial Infarction[4]

The objective of this study is to evaluate the ability of ECGI to noninvasively locate and characterize abnormal cardiac EP substrates during sinus rhythm. It is extremely important to identify the existence of such substrates in patients before they have a major arrhythmic event that can lead to sudden cardiac death. Here we examine this possibility in the context of myocardial infarction, a remodeling process that can produce a highly arrhythmogenic substrate.

A combination of experimental and modeling approaches were used in this study. Epicardial potentials were recorded with a 490-electrode sock from an open-chest dog. Recordings were obtained from a normal heart (control) and from the same heart 2 hours after left anterior descending (LAD) coronary artery occlusion and ethanol injection to create an infarct. This procedure allowed us to use the heart as its own control and to compare epicardial potentials, electrograms, and isochrones pre- and postinfarction in the same heart. Body surface potentials were generated from the measured epicardial potentials in a computer model of the human torso. Realistic geometry errors and measurement noise were added to the torso data to simulate the clinical situation. The perturbed body surface potentials were then used to noninvasively compute epicardial potentials, electrograms and isochrones on the epicardial surface of the heart. The methodology that we have used for the noninvasive reconstruction was described in detail previously.[1-3]

Figure 1 (top row) shows torso potentials, measured epicardial potentials, and noninvasively reconstructed epicardial potentials for the control preinfarction heart at 48 ms (left) and 65 ms (right) after right atrial pacing. The bottom row shows corresponding potentials from the infarcted heart. The 48 ms map clearly shows the localized minimum (white) on the right ventricle (RV) generated by right ventricular epicardial breakthrough (RVBT). Since the right ventricle is not affected by the LAD occlusion and left ventricular (LV) infarction, the RVBT minimum appears in both the control and infarcted hearts. A comparison of LV potentials in the pre- and postinfarcted hearts at 48 ms shows the formation of a large region of negative potential over the infarcted LV area (light gray). This region of negativity results from lack of activation in the underlying necrotic tissue which cannot support normal excitation spread from endocardium to epicardium. The activation front of such spread generates positive potentials on the epicardium;[6] in its absence, negative potentials are generated by more remote fronts propagating away from the infarct. Importantly, both the extensive negative region over the LV infarct and the RVBT epicardial minimum are successfully reconstructed by the noninvasive ECGI from

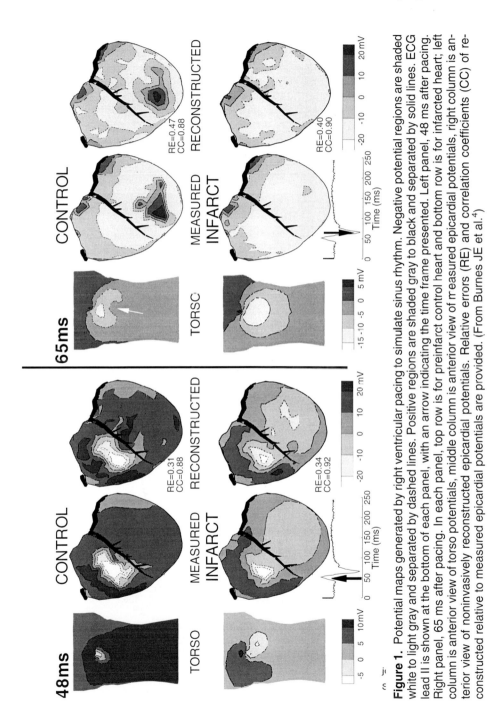

Figure 1. Potential maps generated by right ventricular pacing to simulate sinus rhythm. Negative potential regions are shaded white to light gray and separated by dashed lines. Positive regions are shaded gray to black and separated by solid lines. ECG lead II is shown at the bottom of each panel, with an arrow indicating the time frame presented. Left panel, 48 ms after pacing. Right panel, 65 ms after pacing. In each panel, top row is for preinfarct control heart and bottom row is for infarcted heart; left column is anterior view of torso potentials, middle column is anterior view of measured epicardial potentials, right column is anterior view of noninvasively reconstructed epicardial potentials. Relative errors (RE) and correlation coefficients (CC) of reconstructed relative to measured epicardial potentials are provided. (From Burnes JE et al.[4])

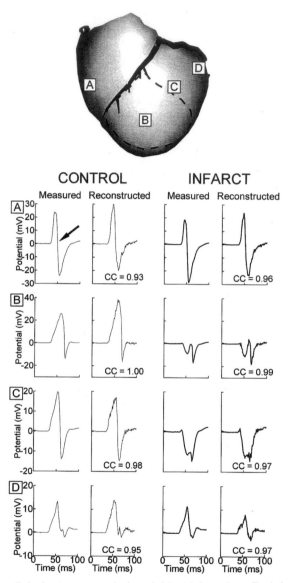

Figure 2. Epicardial electrograms during right atrial pacing. Preinfarction (control) electrograms on left and postinfarction electrograms on right. In each panel, measured electrograms and noninvasively reconstructed electrograms are shown in left and right column, respectively. Arrow in panel A points to intrinsic deflection. (From Burnes JE et al.[4])

the torso potentials (compare reconstructed and measured epicardial potentials at 48 ms, bottom row).

At 65 ms, an island of positive potentials (dark) appears on the LV epicardium of the control heart, reflecting late activation of this LV free wall
region. These positive potentials do not develop in the infarcted heart, indicating that the tissue in this region has become electrically inactive due
to the infarct. Again, ECGI accurately captures the LV region of positive
epicardial potentials in the preinfarction heart and its disappearance in
the infarcted heart.

Figure 2 shows selected electrograms from four representative epicardial sites in the preinfarction (control, left columns) and postinfarction
(infarct, right columns) hearts. For each case, measured electrograms are
on the left and noninvasively reconstructed electrograms on the right. Site
A is located on the RV, sites B and C are over the LV infarcted region, and
site D is on the anterior basal LV away from the infarct. Electrograms from
the preinfarcted heart show the normal RS morphology with a sharp intrinsic deflection (downslope, arrow in A) indicating local activation. The
electrograms from the infarcted heart show changes from control in sites
B and C which lie over the infarct. In site B, the R wave disappears and the
electrogram assumes a negative Q-wave morphology on which a small but
sharp RS deflection is superimposed. The large slow Q-wave envelope is
typical of recordings over infarcted tissue and reflects far-field activity of
wavefronts spreading away from the infarct. The superimposed RS deflection reflects local activation of a small island of surviving myocardium
within the infarct substrate, close to the recording site. Sites A and D do
not change due to the infarct and, being away from the infarcted region,
maintain their RS morphology. Site C is located at the border of the infarct
and shows a small initial R-wave (due to viable tissue bordering the infarct) followed by a large, slow negative Q-wave. The small sharp down-
stroke near the negative peak may reflect local activity of viable tissue
within the infarct region. Note that all of these properties, including the
RS control electrograms, the alteration to slow Q-wave electrograms at
sites over the infarct with superimposed small local deflections, the small
R-wave at the infarct border, and the preservation of RS morphology at locations remote to the infarct are faithfully reconstructed by noninvasive
ECGI.

Imaging Reentrant Activation During Ventricular Tachycardia[5]

The objective of this study is to evaluate the ability of ECGI to noninvasively image reentrant cardiac arrhythmias. A similar combination of
experimental and modeling approaches to that in the previous section is

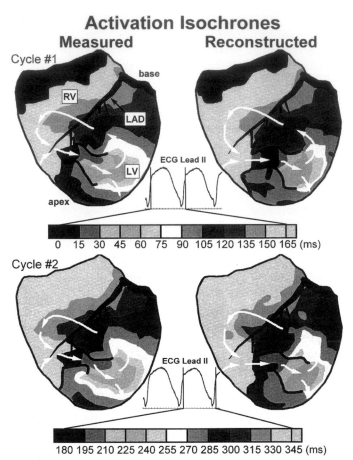

Figure 3. Anterior view of activation isochrones during 2 cycles of ventricular tachycardia (VT). Gray-scale represents times in ms. The right ventricle (RV), left anterior descending (LAD), and left ventricle (LV) are labeled. Lines of block are drawn in black. ECG lead II is shown, with vertical lines indicating time frames displayed for each cycle. Top, first VT cycle. Bottom, second VT cycle. Left, measured isochrones. Right, noninvasively reconstructed isochrones. Arrows indicate direction of wavefront propagation. (From Burns et al.[5] An animated version is available in the research section of www.cwru.edu/med/CBRTC.)

utilized, except that myocardial infarction is produced by 4-day LAD occlusion. The resulting infarct is characterized by a thin epicardial rim of surviving myocardium ("the infarct border zone") which confines reentry circuits during arrhythmic activity to the epicardial surface. Ventricular tachycardia is induced by programmed electrical stimulation.

Figure 3 shows activation isochrones during the arrhythmia for two sequential reentrant beats (cycle #1 on top, cycle #2 on bottom). Measured isochrones are shown on the left and reconstructed isochrones on the right. The activation pattern is a double-loop reentry (arrows), with lines of conduction block (black lines) defining a central common pathway (CCP) in the region of the infarct. The activation front enters the CCP from its basal end, exits at the apical end and divides into two arms that form the two reentry loops. The upper wavefront propagates counterclockwise around the superior line of block toward the base. The lower wavefront propagates clockwise and posterior around the inferior line of block. Crowding of isochrones at the exit from the CCP indicates slowing of conduction as the wavefronts turn around the pivot points at the end of the lines of block. The two wavefronts rejoin at the entrance to the CCP to begin the next reentry cycle of the VT. The noninvasively reconstructed isochrones show the same activation sequence, capturing the reentry loops, the lines of block, the CCP and VT exit site, and the slowing of conduction around pivot points at the tips of the lines of block. Thus, ECGI captures the morphology of the reentrant circuits and its key components during VT.

Figure 4 shows torso potentials and the corresponding (measured and reconstructed) epicardial potentials at three time instants during the VT. The epicardial potential distributions provide another method, complementary to the isochrones of Figure 3, for mapping the reentrant circuit. At 5 ms (panel A), the wavefront enters the CCP while the previous cycle terminates over the basal RV. This is reflected in the positive potential regions at the opening of the CCP and over the basal RV, which are separated by a large negative region. At 50 ms (panel B), the wavefront has exited the CCP and propagated inferiorly, as reflected in the large magnitude positive region and steep potential gradients (indicating the location of the wavefront) over the inferior LV. At 105 ms (panel C), the two arms of the reentry loops are formed and start to envelope the CCP. The reconstructed epicardial potentials closely resemble the measured potentials for all time instances and capture the progression of the wavefront. Note that in panel C, the torso potentials show a smooth and simple pattern with only a single anterior negative region. This pattern does not reflect the complexity of the underlying epicardial pattern which captures the two reentry arms. Despite the lack of detail in the torso potentials, ECGI reconstructs the complexity of the epicardial potentials from the low resolution torso pattern and captures the two forming arms of the reentry circuit.

Conclusions

The studies presented here demonstrate the feasibility of noninvasive reconstructions of abnormal arrhythmogenic substrates and of the activation sequences during cardiac arrhythmias. The ability to noninvasively detect, locate, and characterize an abnormal electrophysiological sub-

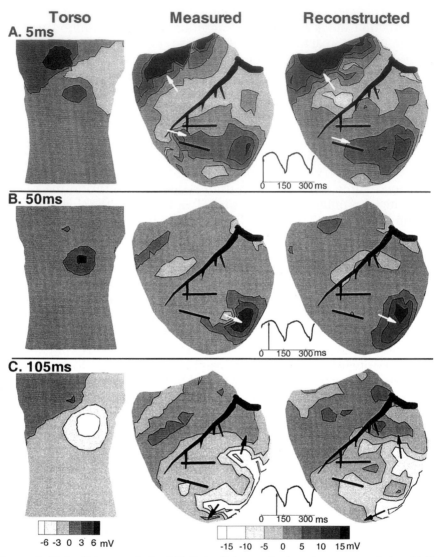

Figure 4. Potential maps during VT. Potentials are displayed as gray scale in mV. Estimated wavefront locations are shown with arrows. A) 5 ms wavefront entering CCP. B) 50 ms wavefront exiting CCP. C) 105 ms wavefront forming arms of reentry circuit. Left to right: torso potentials, measured epicardial potentials, reconstructed epicardial potentials. ECG lead II is shown with arrow indicating time frame presented. (From Burns et al.[5])

strate during sinus rhythm is of important clinical significance because the information can be used to identify patients at risk of developing life-threatening arrhythmias and to guide strategies for prevention. The demonstrated ability of ECGI to reconstruct small inflections generated by islands of surviving myocardium in the infarct is important. Their presence is indicative of the "patchiness" and heterogeneity of the substrate and therefore of the vulnerability to arrhythmia which increases with such nonuniformities of electrical properties.

Noninvasive mapping of the reentry pathway and localization of its critical regions (such as the CCP and exit site) is a prerequisite for guiding noninvasive therapeutic intervention. Once a target is identified and localized, focused energy could be applied for noninvasive ablation. ECGI could also be used to noninvasively image reentrant circuit changes caused by drug administration. It can also guide optimal placement of implantable cardioverter-defibrillator leads or of ablation in the invasive management of arrhythmias.

The experimental strategy in the studies summarized here is to use epicardial potentials recorded in situ with high resolution (490 electrodes) to compute torso potentials, which after contamination by realistic measurement and geometrical errors, serve as the imput data for the noninvasive ECGI reconstructions. In recent experiments we have used measured (rather than computed) body surface potentials as the ECGI noninvasive data, to more closely represent the clinical situation. In the recent experiments, an infarcted dog heart (4-day LAD occlusion) was placed in a human shaped torso-tank, similar to our earlier studies in normal hearts.[1,2] Simultaneous measurement of epicardial potentials provided a gold-standard for direct evaluation of the results. In this setting, ECGI was able to reconstruct the abnormal electrophysiological substrate of the infarct and the activation sequences during reentrant VT with similar accuracy to that reported here. This recent study has been submitted for publication.

References

1. Oster HS, Taccardi B, Lux RL, et al. Noninvasive electrocardiographic imaging: Reconstruction of epicardial potentials, electrograms and isochrones, and localization of single and multiple electrocardiac events. *Circulation* 1997; 96:1012–1024.
2. Oster HS, Taccardi B, Lux RL, et al. Electrocardiographic imaging: Noninvasive characterization of intramural myocardial activation from inverse reconstructed epicardial potentials and electrograms. *Circulation* 1998;97: 1496–1507.
3. Rudy Y, Oster HS. The Electrocardiographic Inverse Problem *CRC Critical Reviews in Biomedical Engineering* 1992;20:25–46.
4. Burnes JE, Taccardi B, MacLeod RS, et al. Noninvasive ECG imaging of electrophysiologically abnormal substrates in infarcted hearts: A model study. *Circulation* 2000;101:533–540.
5. Burnes JE, Taccardi B, Rudy Y. A noninvasive imaging modality for cardiac arrhythmias. *Circulation* 2000;102:2152–2158.
6. Rudy Y. The Electrocardiogram and Cardiac Excitation. In Sperelakis N, Kurachi Y, Terzic A, et al. (eds). **Heart Physiology and Pathophysiology 4th edition**. San Diego, California: Academic Press;2000:133–148.

Chapter 6

Spatial Gradients in Activation Frequency:
A Mechanism of Stable Ventricular Fibrillation

José Jalife, MD, Faramarz H. Samie, PhD,
Jacques Beaumont, PhD

Introduction

Ventricular fibrillation (VF) is the most important cardiac electrical derangement leading to sudden cardiac death, but its mechanisms remains unknown. Prevailing hypotheses today to explain such mechanisms include: 1) the multiple wavelet hypothesis,[1] 2) spiral/scroll breakup,[2,3] and 3) single high-frequency rotor with fibrillatory conduction.[4] From ECG recordings, VF is visualized as exceedingly complex and turbulent electrical activity, which is consistent with both the multiple wavelet reentry and spiral breakup conjectures. However, neither mechanism can account for the organized activity documented in VF by a number of authors.[5,6] Moreover, recent data show that fibrillatory conduction from a dominant high frequency source may underlie VF in the rabbit heart[7,8] and in the isolated sheep ventricular preparations.[9] Those studies demonstrated that rapidly succeeding wavefronts emanating from reentrant sources propagate throughout the ventricles giving rise to wavelets and intermittently blocking at specific locations, thus forming dominant frequency (DF) domains. As such, fibrillatory conduction can account for the complex patterns of wavefront propagation as well as the organized activity documented in VF.

[1] This work is supported in part by grants PO1 HL39707 and RO1 HL60843 from the National Heart and Blood Institute, National Institutes of Health.

From Virag N, Blanc O, Kappenberger L (eds): *Computer Simulation and Experimental Assessment of Cardiac Electrophysiology.* ©Futura Publishing Co., Inc., Armonk, NY, 2001.

Here we discuss recent results of video imaging experiments in which a voltage sensitive dye (Di-4-ANEPPS) was used to study organization of activity during VF in the isolated Langendorff-perfused guinea pig heart.[10] The video images (typically ~4100 pixels) were acquired at ~600 frames per second with an effective spatial resolution of > 0.4 mm. Fast Fourier transform (FFT) was applied to the 2.3-second segments of the optical signal from each pixel of the epicardial image, which provided a spectral resolution of 0.47 Hz. The position of the largest spectral peak (DF) was determined for each pixel, and color maps of spatial DF distribution were constructed for each recording of VF.

Spatial Frequency Gradients During Ventricular Fibrillation

As illustrated in the left panel of Figure 1, the DF maps of VF appeared surprisingly simple. They consisted of few relatively large areas ("domains") of uniform DF. A major part of the epicardial surface of the anterior wall of the left ventricle was occupied by a continuous domain with a DF of 26.7 Hz. Analysis of the optical signal in this domain revealed a relatively stable rotor (data not shown) that underwent as many as 150 rotations at a stable period of 37.5 ms; i.e., frequency of 26.7 Hz.

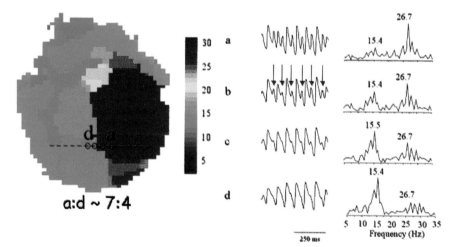

Figure 1. High-resolution frequency analysis of ventricular fibrillation in the Langendorff-perfused guinea pig heart. The left panel is a representative color map of dominant frequencies (DFs). The highest frequency domain (red) on the anterior free wall of the left ventricle corresponds to 26.7 Hz (color bar indicates frequency in Hz). The DFs in the right ventricle range between 12 and 15.5 Hz. Individual a–d pixel recordings and their corresponding frequency spectra show transition in frequencies from left to right ventricles at the boundaries between domains along the horizontal line a–d on the map. Red arrows on trace b indicate 2:1 block from a to b.

The highest frequency domain was surrounded by lower frequency domains which, as shown in Figure 1, established a DF gradient from the left ventricle (LV) to the right ventricle (RV) and from the anterior to the posterior walls (data not shown). This gradient was the result of the occurrence of spatially distributed intermittent block processes occurring at the boundaries between domains, which resulted in an overall pattern of fibrillatory conduction. The analysis of activation pattern across a boundary between the highest frequency domain in the LV and an adjacent domain along a horizontal line (a–d) across the left anterior descending artery on the ventricular wall is presented on the right panel of Figure 1. Single pixel recordings and their respective power spectra show the gradual transformation of the local activity as the high frequency wavefronts attempted to propagate from the left to the right ventricle. Arrows indicate the occurrence of intermittent conduction block between points a and d. Spectra a through d reveal reciprocal changes of the amplitude of two main peaks, with a gradual transition from 26.7 to 15.4 Hz. Similar results were obtained in 10 experiments.

The data illustrated in Figure 1 provide the first demonstration that, during VF, the LV anterior free wall is the preferred location of a stable reentrant source that activates the ventricles at 25–32 Hz (i.e., from 1500 to as much as 1920 rotations/min!). Moreover, the results also show that wave propagation away from this stable high frequency reentrant source is complicated by the formation of wave breaks and intermittent conduction block. Thus, it is clear from these results that somehow the LV is capable of sustaining 1:1 propagation at such astonishingly high frequencies. However, the right ventricle is not, which suggests that there are substantial electrophysiological differences between both ventricles, which are relatively small at slow frequencies, but become clearly manifest during the high frequencies associated with VF.

APD Abbreviation and Rapid Rotation Frequency

During VF in the guinea pig heart, the local activation cycle length (~ 30 ms) is significantly briefer than the guinea pig cardiac action potential duration (~ 200 ms), when measured at constant stimulation frequencies of 1 Hz.[11] Recent computer simulations suggest that the activation at extremely fast rates by a rotor may be the result of the strong repolarizing influence exerted by the center of rotation (core), which as shown in Figure 2, abbreviates the action potential duration (APD) of cells in its immediate surroundings. However, with increasing distance from the core, this influence weakens and the APD progressively increases, up to a distance of 1 cm.[12] Consequently, the tissue close to the core achieves very fast cycle lengths, whereas far from the core, the myocardium cannot conduct all

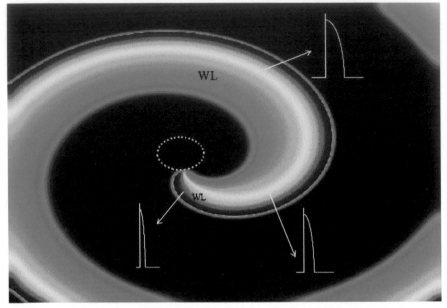

Figure 2. Sustained reentrant activity in a 2 cm by 2 cm sheet of modified Luo & Rudy I model cells (for details of model parameters see ref 12). Note the spatial distribution of wavelength (WL) and action potential duration from the center to the periphery of the rotating wave. The wavefront is in red and resting tissue appears in dark blue. The dotted circle indicates the position of the core.

the impulses emanating from the rotor at such high rates. The ultimate result is fibrillatory conduction with highly nonuniform distribution of multiple broken waves, particularly at the boundaries between domains.[9,10] In theory, this effect may provide a basis for the gradient in DFs observed in the guinea pig ventricles during VF (Figure 1). Nevertheless, while this mechanism may account for the shortening of the APD and the formation of DF domains, it does not explain the consistent localization of the fastest DF domain to the anterior free wall of the LV.

The mechanism responsible for stabilization of the rotor in the LV remains to be determined. Recently Kim et al.[13] suggested that the source-sink mismatch created by the geometrical arrangement of the papillary muscles with respect to the ventricular wall may serve as site of rotor anchoring. Thus, in the context of their finding, the 2 papillary muscles present in the LV of the guinea pig, one near the LV apex and the other in the LV anterior free wall, may conceivably play a role in the stabilization of the reentrant circuit. However, in contrast to the experiments of Kim et al.,[13] in which they noted that the reentrant circuits often terminated by the other wavelets that exist during VF, we observed that the reentrant source may remain stable within the field of view for approximately 150 rotations. Nevertheless, at this point one cannot rule out the possibility that the papillary muscles present in the LV of the guinea pig heart and the source-sink mismatch that they create plays a role in the stabilization of the reentrant circuit.

An alternative explanation for the stabilization of the rotor in the LV is provided by recent preliminary experiments from our laboratory showing a difference in the conductance of the background current of the cells in the RV and the LV, particularly at potentials positive to the resting membrane potential.[10] During normal propagation, the wavetail follows the wavefront after the delayed rectifier current (I_K) is triggered, which rapidly repolarizes the cell.[12] In contrast, during reentry, APD is significantly abbreviated and repolarization occurs via I_{K1} and the electrotonically mediated influence of the core.[12] Computer simulations show that in addition to controlling the APD, the large I_{K1} stabilizes the vortex by reducing the wavefront-tail interaction whereas I_{K1} reduction produces a drift in the vortex.[12] Thus, it is conceivable that the larger amplitude of the background conductance that we have observed in the LV[10] may stabilize the rotor and the high frequency domains in the LV by reducing the APD near the core, subsequently leading to a decrease in the degree of wavefront wavetail interactions. Work from our laboratory utilizing a combination of optical mapping, patch clamping, computer modeling and molecular biology techniques is currently in progress to determine the potential role of spatial gradients in potassium ion channel density and distribution in the mechanism of high-frequency rotor stabilization in the LV with fibrillatory conduction toward the RV.

Conclusions

Gradients in excitation frequency and fibrillatory conduction have been shown to exist between the left and right sides of the heart both during atrial fibrillation in the sheep heart[14] and ventricular fibrillation in the pig.[15] However, to our knowledge, there is no precedent for the demonstration of a highly consistent localization of the rotor on the anterior free wall of the LV, and there is also no precedent for the reproducible localization of the wavebreaks around that rotor. Moreover, the demonstration of a strong correlation between the maintenance of fibrillation and its stationary left-to-right gradients of excitation frequency is completely new. Most importantly, the possibility that differences in ionic current density between myocytes in the right and the left ventricle may explain the data in the whole heart, suggests unambiguously a molecular basis for the formation of a stable rotor in the LV and for fibrillatory conduction toward the RV.

In summary, in the isolated guinea pig heart, a single stable source within the LV free wall may be the underlying mechanism of VF, and possibly the localization of the rotor may be the consequence of the underlying electrophysiological properties of the tissue, i.e., differential distribution of ion channels. Importantly, work discussed here strongly suggests that the fragmentation of wavelets emanating from a high frequency source may be a general phenomenon, i.e., species independent, and that the frequency of rotor may be the critical factor in determining whether fragmentation and new wavelet formation occurs in the heart.

References

1. Moe GK. On the multiple wavelet hypothesis of atrial fibrillation. *Archives Internationales de Pharmacodynamie et de Therapie* 1962;CXL:183–188.
2. Fenton F, Karma A. Vortex dynamics in three-dimensional continuous myocardium with fiber rotation: Filament instability and fibrillation. *Chaos* 1998;8:20–47.
3. Panfilov AV. Spiral breakup as a model of ventricular fibrillation. *Chaos* 1998; 8:57–64.
4. Jalife J, Berenfeld O, Skanes A, et al. Mechanisms of atrial fibrillation: Mother rotors or multiple daughter wavelets, or both? *J Cardiovasc Electrophysiol* 1998;9:S2–12.
5. Damle RS, Kanaan NM, Robinson NS, et al. Spatial and temporal linking of epicardial activation directions during ventricular fibrillation in dogs. Evidence for underlying organization. *Circulation* 1992;86:1547–1558.
6. Rogers JM, Huang J, Smith WM, et al. Incidence, evolution, and spatial distribution of functional reentry during ventricular fibrillation in pigs. *Cir Res* 1999;84:945–954.
7. Chen J, Mandapati R, Berenfeld O, et al. High-frequency periodic sources underlie ventricular fibrillation in the isolated rabbit heart. *Circ Res* 2000; 86:86–93.
8. Samie FH, Mandapati R, Gray RA, et al. A mechanism of transition from ventricular fibrillation to tachycardia: Effect of calcium channel blockade on the dynamics of rotating waves. *Circ Res* 2000;86:684–691.
9. Zaitsev AV, Berenfeld O, Mironov SF, et al. Distribution of excitation frequencies on the epicardial and endocardial surfaces of fibrillating ventricular wall of the sheep heart. *Circ Res* 2000;86:408–417.
10. Samie FH, Berenfeld O, Mironov SF, et al. An ionic mechanism for ventricular fibrillation in the Langendorff-perfused guinea pig heart. *Circulation* 2000;102(II):341. Abstract.
11. Priori SG, Napolitano C, Cantu F, et al. Differential response to Na+ channel blockade, beta-adrenergic stimulation, and rapid pacing in a cellular model mimicking the SCN5A and HERG defects present in the long-QT syndrome. *Circ Res* 1996;78:1009–1015.
12. Beaumont J, Davidenko N, Davidenko JM, et al. Spiral waves in two-dimensional models of ventricular muscle: Formation of a stationary core. *Biophys J* 1998;75:1–14.

13. Kim YH, Yashima M, Wu TJ, et al. Mechanism of procainamide-induced prevention of spontaneous wave break during ventricular fibrillation. Insight into the maintenance of fibrillation wave fronts. *Circulation* 1999;100:666–674.
14. Berenfeld O, Mandapati R, Dixit S, et al. Spatially distributed dominant excitation frequencies reveal hidden organization in atrial fibrillation in the Langendorff-perfused sheep heart. *J Cardiovasc Electrophysiol* 2000;11(8): 869–879.
15. Newton JC, Evans FG, Chattipakorn N, et al. Peak frequency distribution across the whole fibrillating heart. *Pacing Clinical Electrophysiol* 2000;23: 617. Part II Abstract.

Chapter 7

Ventricular Excitation: Wavefronts, Electrograms and Potential Patterns

Piero Colli-Franzone, PhD

Introduction

We present a brief summary of the methodological approach for large-scale simulations of the excitation sequences, potential patterns and electrograms developed using a macroscopic analysis based on the bidomain model.

Macroscopic Anisotropic Bidomain Model

In the macroscopic bidomain representation of the cardiac tissue, the anisotropic structure of the two averaged continuous media (intra and the extracellular) is characterized by means of the conductivity tensors M_i and M_e. These tensors are related to the structure of the cardiac fibers and the local macroscopic conductivity coefficients $\sigma_l^{i,e} \sigma_t^{i,e}$ measured along and across the local fiber direction, and assuming axial symmetry, are given by $M_{i,e}(\mathbf{x}) = \sigma_t^{i,e} I + (\sigma_l^{i,e} - \sigma_t^{i,e})\mathbf{a}(\mathbf{x})\mathbf{a}^T(\mathbf{x})$ with $\mathbf{a}(\mathbf{x})$ the local fiber direction.

Imposing the conservation of currents, i.e., that the exchange between the two media must balance the membrane current flow per unit volume, one derives a reaction-diffusion system defined in the cardiac tissue. Denoting $\mathbf{J}_i = -M_i \nabla u_i$, $\mathbf{J}_e = -M_e \nabla u_e$ the intra and extracellular current densities, in terms of the intra and extracellular potentials $u_i(\mathbf{x},t)$, $u_e(\mathbf{x},t)$, a singular perturbation structure becomes evident when writing

From Virag N, Blanc O, Kappenberger L (eds): *Computer Simulation and Experimental Assessment of Cardiac Electrophysiology.* ©Futura Publishing Co., Inc., Armonk, NY, 2001.

the Reaction-Diffusion (R-D) system in a suitable dimensionless form (singular perturbation structure):

$$\partial_t \begin{bmatrix} 1 & -1 \\ -1 & 1 \end{bmatrix} \begin{pmatrix} u_i \\ u_e \end{pmatrix} - \varepsilon \begin{bmatrix} \text{div } M_i \nabla & 0 \\ 0 & \text{div } M_e \nabla \end{bmatrix} \begin{pmatrix} u_i \\ u_e \end{pmatrix} + \frac{1}{\varepsilon} \begin{pmatrix} i_{ion} \\ -i_{ion} \end{pmatrix} = 0 \quad (1)$$

where the dimensionless parameter $\varepsilon \approx 10^{-3} \div 10^{-2}$. We are in presence of a slow diffusion and fast reaction; moreover the coupling between the two equations is done through the temporal term which displays a degenerated structure. A qualitative macroscopic description of the excitation phase in a normal ventricle was achieved by deriving the asymptotic behavior of the traveling wavefront solutions of the R-D system. In fact the singular structure allows the development of a propagating excitation interface associated to a fast transition of the transmembrane potential $v(\mathbf{x},t) = u_i(\mathbf{x},t) - u_e(\mathbf{x},t)$ from the resting to the excited value. This qualitative macro-analysis was developed under the following assumptions:

- cardiac tissue is fully recovered;
- ionic membrane current is instantaneous and described by a cubic-like function $i_{ion} = F(v)$ having as zeros the values for rest, threshold and plateau v_r, v_{th}, v_p.

During the excitation phase the potential v exhibits a monotonic time behavior and if we introduce the activation time $\varphi(\mathbf{x})$ as the time instant at which $v(\mathbf{x},\varphi(\mathbf{x})) = (v_r + v_p)/2$, then the excitation wavefront $S_\varepsilon(t)$ is given by the surface level of the activation time, i.e., $S_\varepsilon(t) = \{\mathbf{x} \in H, \quad \varphi(\mathbf{x}) = t\}$, where H represents the heart tissue.

Motion of the Excitation Wavefront

The intra and extra conductivity coefficients along the direction ξ are given by $\sigma_{i,e}(\mathbf{x},\xi) = \xi^T M_{i,e}(\mathbf{x}) \xi$ with $\xi^T \xi = 1$. Based on this, we define the anisotropic indicatrix:

$$\Phi(x,\xi) = \sqrt{\sigma(\mathbf{x},\xi)} = \sqrt{\frac{\sigma_i(\mathbf{x},\xi)\sigma_e(\mathbf{x},\xi)}{\sigma_i(\mathbf{x},\xi) + \sigma_e(\mathbf{x},\xi)}} \quad (2)$$

In the eikonal approach the wavefront $S_\varepsilon(t)$ moves along the Euclidean normal direction $\mathbf{n}$ with a velocity $\theta_\varepsilon(\mathbf{x},\mathbf{n})$ given by (excitation wavefront motion):

$$\theta_\varepsilon(\mathbf{x},\mathbf{n}) = \Phi(\mathbf{x},\mathbf{n})(c - \varepsilon \text{ div}\Phi_\xi(\mathbf{x},\mathbf{n})) + O(\varepsilon^2) \quad (3)$$

Anisotropic geometric evolution laws of this type are also called eikonal-curvature models since the term $\kappa_\phi = $ div Φ_ξ $(\mathbf{x,n})$ represents the anisotropic *mean* curvature in a suitable Finsler metric.[1] The parameter c is related to the asymptotic velocity of the action potential traveling in an infinite cable. In term of the activation time $\varphi(x)$ the velocity is given by θ_ε $(\mathbf{x,n}) = 1/|\nabla\varphi|$. Moreover, since the propagating front is described in a Cartesian representation, it is more convenient for computational purposes to use the following equation, which is equivalent to Equation (3) except for the second order terms in ε:

$$-\varepsilon \text{ div } [\Phi(\mathbf{x}, \nabla\phi)\Phi_\xi (\mathbf{x}, \nabla\varphi) + c \ \Phi(x, \nabla\varphi) = 1 + O(\varepsilon^2) \qquad (4)$$

We remark that the activation time $\varphi(x)$ is a smooth function. Therefore the numerical simulation of the eikonal model can be performed on a quasi-uniform grid with a spatial step greater than 1–2 mm. This allows a strong reduction of the computational complexity for large-scale simulations with respect to the R-D system. Numerical simulations showed that the eikonal model reproduces the qualitative features of the excitation sequences elicited by pacing the ventricular wall in exposed dog heart experiments.

We validated the general rules describing the propagation and the shape of the excitation fronts by simulating some excitation sequences. We applied a local stimulus to an ellipsoidal ventricular model with intramural fiber rotation, fiber obliqueness in the epi- endocardial direction and with the presence of a network of Purkinje ventricular junctions. We pointed out two anisotropic features of the spread of excitation, i.e., the excitation return pathways toward the pacing level.[2] The transmural fiber rotation creates these excitation pathways, starting from the pacing site, first proceeding away from it and then turning back, bending and pointing towards the myocardial level from which the excitation was first delivered (see left panel of Figure 1). An effect of the intramural fiber rotation is to produce a transverse acceleration of the parts of the wavefront propagating across fibers; at several centimeters from the pacing site, they exhibit a dimple-like inflection (see the right panel of Figure 2).

The knowledge of $v(x,t)$ allows us to simulate the time-space extracellular potential on the QRS complex. The numerical approximation of the differential equation in terms of (u_e, v) allows the use of the same quasi-uniform grid as considered for the eikonal model. This grid with a coarse mesh size leads to fairly accurate results at a distance from the excitation layers and has been used to simulate the main features of the patterns displayed by the extracellular potential maps.[2] In order to simulate a relatively small number of electrograms (EGs) free from numerical artifacts, the differential representation is not convenient since it requires a

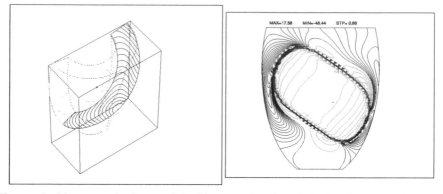

Figure 1. Monoventricular model with central epicardial stimulation. Left panel: isochrone map depicting the spread of excitation on the diagonal intramural surface; time interval between successive isochrones is 5 msec. Right panel: epicardial potential map at 45 msec after pacing.

sequence of meshes with dynamical tracking of the propagating excitation layers. This is not an easy task in a 3D environment. Therefore, for the computation of the integral on H, we used a *fixed adaptive mesh* around the singularity at the observation point $\mathbf{x}$ coupled with an *adaptive sub-element techniques* for the elements near or inside the excitation layer.[3] Denoting by M_0 and u_0 the conductivity tensor and the potential in the extra-

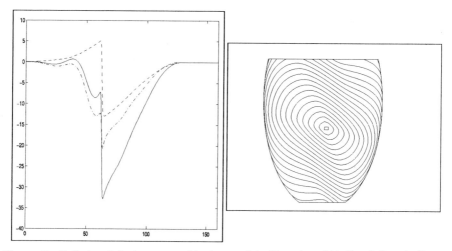

Figure 2. Fully insulated monoventricular model with epicardial stimulation. Left pannel: superimposed components of the split form of electrogram at the site marked by a dot; the full, axial and conormal electrograms are displayed as continuous, dash-dot and dashed lines respectively. Right pannel: isochrone map depicting the spread of excitation on the epicardial surface.

cardiac domain we set:

$$\hat{M} = \begin{cases} M_i\,(\mathbf{x}) + M_e\,(\mathbf{x}) \\ M_0\,(\mathbf{x}) \end{cases} \quad u(\mathbf{x},t) = \begin{cases} u_e\,(\mathbf{x},t) & \mathbf{x} \in H \\ u_0\,(\mathbf{x},t) & \mathbf{x} \in \Omega, \end{cases} \quad \mathbf{J}_v\,(\mathbf{x},t) = -M_i\,\nabla v(\mathbf{x},t)$$

(5)

where Ω represents the extra-cardiac domain. From the current conservation law we can deduct the following integral representation for EGs:[3]

$$\omega(\mathbf{x},t) = u(\mathbf{x},t) - \frac{1}{|\partial H_{epi}|} \int_{\partial H_{epi}} u(\xi,t)d\sigma_\xi = \int_H \mathbf{J}_v^T\,\nabla_\xi \psi\,(\xi,\mathbf{x})d\xi \qquad (6)$$

where H_{epi} represents the epicardium and the Green function ψ satisfies a suitable elliptic problem with a singularity at the observation point $\mathbf{x}$. One of the boundary conditions imposed for the "*lead field*" ψ reflects that the potential field $\omega(\mathbf{x},t)$ has a zero average on the epicardium ∂H_{epi}. Experimental observations with isolated canine hearts in a torso-shaped tank showed that the potential at Wilson's central terminal is close to the potential averaged on the tank and on the epicardial surface.

General Rules Describing the Potential Maps and Electrograms

Potential maxima are invariably facing the intramural portion of the wavefronts moving mainly along fibers and create a far-field positivity throughout the thickness of the wall on the epi- and the endocardial surfaces. Moreover the positive equipotential lines surrounding the maxima exhibit an expanding C-shape which subsequently undergoes a stretching and bending (see right panel of Figure1).

Concerning the epicardial EGs, when applying an epicardial pacing we observe a biphasic waveform for sites reached by the wavefront along fibers, while for sites across fiber EGs display a mono to tetra or penta-phasic waveshape with the presence of humps followed by spikes (see Figure 3). Moreover the EG intrinsic deflections cover a wide range. We first identified in the reference potential the origin of the shift of the R-S extracellular jump, whose excursion ranged between an almost negative to an almost positive potential value. This drift of the reference potential introduces a positive trend creating or emphasizing R waves, humps and spikes. For locations near the epicardial pacing site, EGs exhibit from a negative jump or a small positive R-wave, to a positive R-wave and a neg-

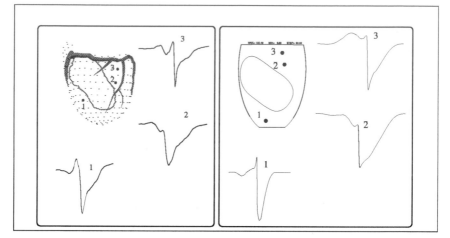

Figure 3. Comparison of measured (left panel) and computed (right panel) epicardial electrograms elicited by central epicardial pacing. The measured and simulated isochrones are indicated on the heart surface at 40 and 45 msec respectively.

ative S-wave of similar magnitude. In the extinction area, EGs exhibit a positive jump with a small negative S-wave.[4]

We investigated the mechanisms that generate polymorphic waveforms using a split form of the cardiac sources. For suitable parameters α, β we have to identify $M_i = \alpha M + \beta \mathbf{aa}^T$, where $M = M_i + M_e$. Based on this formulation, the impressed or source current $\mathbf{J}_v(\mathbf{x},t)$ can be decomposed into the sum of two dipolar current densities, with axes parallel to the conormal vector $M\nabla v$ and to the fiber direction $\mathbf{a}$ respectively:

$$\mathbf{J}_v = -M_i\nabla v = \mathbf{J}_c + \mathbf{J}_a, \quad \mathbf{J}_c = -\alpha M\nabla v, \quad \mathbf{J}_a = -\beta(\mathbf{a}^T\nabla v)\mathbf{a} \qquad (7)$$

The associated potential field is then split into the conormal and axial field components ω_c, ω_a given by:

$$\omega(\mathbf{x},t) = \omega_c + \omega_a, \quad \omega_c(\mathbf{x},t) = \int_H \mathbf{J}_c^T \nabla_\xi \psi d\xi, \quad \omega_a(\mathbf{x},t) = \int_H \mathbf{J}_a^T \nabla_\xi \psi d\xi \qquad (8)$$

The split form of the cardiac sources provides an explanation of the origin of humps and spikes appearing in the multiphasic QRS waveforms. The left panel of Figure 2 displays the EGs components and we can see that the conormal EG exhibits a biphasic waveshape while a multiphasic behavior can be mainly attributed to the axial component. Since for a bidomain with equal anisotropy ratio we have $\beta = 0$, the full EG $\omega(\mathbf{x},t)$ reduces to the biphasic conormal EG $\omega_c(\mathbf{x},t)$. Therefore polymorphic waveshapes are mainly an effect of the axial sources, i.e. of an unequal anisotropic bidomain.

Limitations and Conclusion

The methodology and analysis described here is confined to the depolarization phase only, but it could be extended to the description of wavefront propagation. Therefore it would be possible to study potential patterns and morphological variety of EGs in ischemic or necrotic tissue in order to detect reliable markers for the localization of the ischemic zones.

References

1. Bellettini G, Colli Franzone P, Paolini M. Convergence of front propagation for anisotropic bistable reaction-diffusion equations. *Asymp Anal* 1997;15: 325–358.
2. Colli Franzone P, Guerri L, Pennacchio M, et al. Spread of excitation in 3-D models of the anisotropic cardiac tissue. II: Effects of fiber architecture and ventricular geometry. III: Effects of ventricular geometry and fiber structure on the potential distribution. *Math Biosci* 1998;147:131–171;151:51–98.
3. Colli Franzone P, Pennacchio M, Guerri L. Accurate computation of electrograms in the left ventricular wall. *Math Mod and Meth in Appl Sci* 2000;10(4):507–538.
4. Colli Franzone P, Pennacchio M, Guerri L, et al. Anisotropic mechanisms for multiphasic unipolar electrograms. Simulation studies and experimental recordings. *Ann Biomed Eng* 2000;28:1–17.

Chapter 8

Three-Dimensional Organization of Reentry in Fibrillating Ventricular Wall

Arkady M. Pertsov, PhD

Introduction

High-resolution mapping studies of polymorphic ventricular tachycardia (PVT) and ventricular fibrillation (VF) in animal models and humans suggest that these arrhythmias are caused by a vortex-like reentrant activity, also known as spiral wave reentry.[1] What is the three-dimensional (3D) organization of the spiral wave reentry in the depth of the ventricular wall?

Scroll Waves and Filaments

The simplest configuration of a 3D rotating wave, the so called simple scroll is shown in Figure 1. The left panels show snapshots of a simple scroll obtained in a computer simulation using a 3D array of electrically coupled excitable cells described by the FitzHugh-Nagumo equations. The rotation of the scroll occurs around a central line (f-f') called the filament. In any section of a scroll perpendicular to the filament the observer will see an identical spiral wave. The right panels show the recordings of the transmembrane potential at different distances from the filament. Cells close to f-f', like those located in the core of a 2D spiral, have very small amplitudes of excitation (see trace 4). These cells, however, are functionally normal and can develop normal action potentials when the filament moves to a different location. The presence of low amplitudes near the

---

From Virag N, Blanc O, Kappenberger L (eds): *Computer Simulation and Experimental Assessment of Cardiac Electrophysiology.* ©Futura Publishing Co., Inc., Armonk, NY, 2001.

center can be used for localization of the core and the filament (see Figure 2). Scroll waves may have different orientations with respect to the epicardial and endocardial surfaces. Figure 1B shows a simple scroll with a filament parallel to the epicardial surface. In this case mapping of both epicardial and endocardial surfaces will not reveal any reentrant activity; only large breakthrough areas will be observed.

Among various possible filament orientations, some are more probable than others. Theoretical studies[2,3] suggest that scroll wave filaments have a tendency to align with the direction of myocardial fibers. Accordingly, by taking into account the fact that myocardial fibers run parallel, or at small angles, to the epicardial surface, one should conclude that the filament orientations parallel to the surface (as in Figure 1B) are more likely than the transmural orientation shown in Figure 1A. This can explain the relatively rare occurrence and instability of spiral wave activity on the ventricular surface during polymorphic ventricular tachycardia and fibrillation.[4] A recent experimental example of arrhythmia that is most likely produced by a concealed scroll wave can be found.[5]

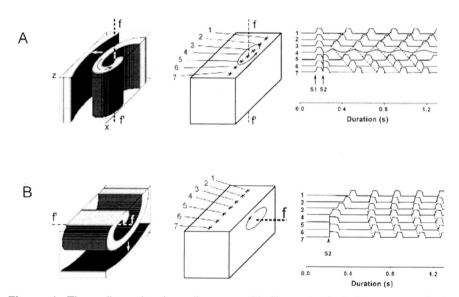

Figure 1. Three-dimensional scroll waves with filament orientations perpendicular (A) and parallel (B) to the surface (adapted from Pertsov et al.[1]). The model consists of an anisotropic ($D_y/D_x=4$) array of $48\times48\times48$ excitable elements connected to each other through a diffusion term. Left panels in A and B show snapshots of a rotating scroll. Non-excited areas are transparent. The rotation axis f-f' (filament) is shown by a dashed line. The white arrow shows the direction of pulse propagation. The scroll waves were initiated by a cross-field stimulation method; the basic (S1) and premature (S2) stimuli were delivered from the front and left lateral surfaces (A) and from the front and bottom surfaces (B). Right panels: Action potentials recorded from the top surface of the cube. Numbers indicate the location of the recording sites in the middle panels, and arrows below the traces indicate the times of stimulation.

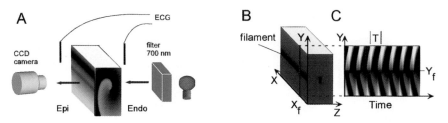

Figure 2. Filament visualization using the transillumination technique (a computer simulation). A) The 3D-block in the center represents a slab of myocardial tissue containing a rotating scroll wave. Gray levels indicate the calculated light intensity. B) Image of the block with the filament projection obtained via time-averaging of sequential frames. C) Time-space plot (Y,T) diagram of a vertical slice X_f with a zigzag pattern indicating the position of the filament in this slice.

Visualization of the Filament

As we show below, scroll waves and their filaments can be visualized using optical methods. Our group has developed and successfully used such methods for the visualization of scroll wave filaments in 3D chemical excitable media.[6] Here we demonstrate that the same approaches can be adapted to the analysis of the scroll waves in the myocardial wall. The idea of these methods is based on using transillumination. The myocardial wall, stained with a voltage sensitive dye, is placed between a light source and a video camera. Changes in the transmembrane voltage produced by a 3D rotating wave of excitation inside the myocardial wall result in variations of light intensity that are recorded by the video camera. The filament, or more accurately its projection, is reconstructed from the computational analysis of the recorded sequence of images.[6]

In our first transillumination experiments in myocardial tissue we utilized a voltage sensitive fluorescent dye (di-4-ANEPPS). We used the ability of myocardial tissue to transmit the red light emitted by the fluorescent dye significantly better than the green excitation light. This property enabled us to reconstruct activation patterns in layers located on the surface and 2 mm below the surface. Figure 3 represents the experimental demonstration of a scroll wave concealed in the thickness of the ventricular wall during sustained tachycardia in coronary-perfused right ventricle of the sheep using this technique.[7]

Recently we were able to implement the transillumination technique in such a way that information not only from the subendocardial and subepicardial layers but from all thickness of the wall could be extracted.[8] The major step involved the replacement of the fluorescent dye with an absorbance dye, RH-155, working in the red range of the spectrum. This eliminated problems caused by poor penetration of the green excitation light through the tissue. Changes in the transmembrane voltage produced

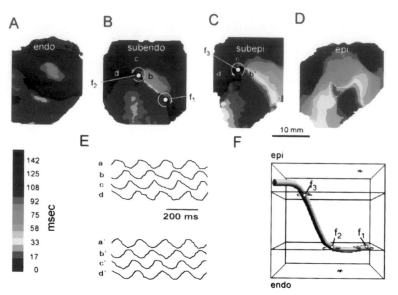

Figure 3. A concealed scroll wave during tachycardia in isolated right ventricular wall. A–D) Isochronal maps recorded from the endocardial, subendocardial, subepicardial, and epicardial layers, respectively using a combination of transillumination and epifluorescence measurements. Circles f_1, f_2 and f_3 show the sites of intersection of the filament with the observation planes. Note that surface layers (A,D) do not show any reentrant activity, yet it can be identified in the intramural (B,C) layers. E) Optical recordings from the individual sites in the subendocardial (B) and subepicardial (C) layers (points a,b,c,d and a′,b′,c′,d′, respectively). Activation sequences clearly show the reentrant activity. F) A hypothetical shape of the filament consistent with the isochronal maps shown in panels A–D. Asterisks indicate the breakthrough sites. Adapted from Pertsov et al.[8]

by a rotating wave of excitation affect the light absorbance of the dye and are recorded by a video camera as variations in transmittance. Each image is a weighted sum of signals coming from all layers and is similar to an optical tomographic projection. By taking a sequence of such images at a rate significantly higher than the rotation frequency, we obtain multiple projections of the same rotating scroll wave. The filament was subsequently visualized by processing of the information contained in these projections using an algorithm described by Vinson et al.[6]

Figure 2 illustrates one of the methods of filament reconstruction in transillumination experiments - the time averaging method.[6] This method makes use of the fact that the immediate neighborhood of the filament is not excited by the circulating excitation wave. In this computational illustration we simulated a 3D block of myocardial tissue with a scroll wave oriented parallel to the surface. Electrical properties were described using the Luo-Rudy equations. The transillumination signal was calculated assuming exponential decay of light intensity inside the wall. In panel A, the spiral and the end of the filament can be seen from the edge of the block. The time averaging of sequential frames over one or more rotation cycles reveals a dark shadow which is the projection of the filament onto the surface of the preparation. The position of the shadow (panel B, center) agrees well with the real filament position. Panel C shows another method of filament reconstruction based on time-space plot analysis.[6] Both methods give consistent results.

Stable Filaments During Ventricular Fibrillation

We used the transillumination technique to study polymorphic ventricular tachycardia and fibrillation. The experiments were conducted on isolated coronary-perfused and superfused right ventricular wall preparations of sheep.[4] VF was induced by rapid pacing. The preparations were stained with the absorbance voltage-sensitive dye RH-155. The variations in transmembrane voltage were detected by measuring light transmittance through the tissue at 700 nm using a high-speed digital CCD video camera. The light source and the camera were located on the endocardial and epicardial sides of the preparation, respectively.

In 6 out of 9 episodes of sustained ventricular tachycardia and ventricular fibrillation we observed stable intramural filaments (usually one, sometimes two) that persisted throughout the whole length of our recording (2 sec) for more than 10–15 cycles. Repetitive recordings obtained every 2–3 minutes often showed the filaments at the same location. Figure 4B shows the stable filament obtained during an episode of VF in sheep right ventricle using the time-averaging method. The filament appears as a dark shadow (arrowheads). No such shadow was present before the initiation of tachycardia and after its termination (Figure 4C). Note that the shadow from the stimulating electrode (star) remains after the termination of arrhythmia. The stability of the filament contrasted strikingly with the

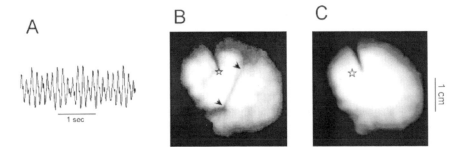

Figure 4. Scroll wave filament in fibrillating right ventricular wall. A) ECG recording of the VF episode. B) Time averaged image of the transillumination signal. Arrowheads show the filament position. C) The same image after defibrillation.

irregularity of the ECG (panel A) and surface activation patterns (not shown).

These findings lead us to hypothesize *that sustained PVT and VF in our experimental model are driven by stable scrolls with filaments concealed in the depth of the myocardial wall.* We assume that the irregularity of the ECG results from complex patterns of local propagation and intermittent block (fibrillatory propagation), which are caused by the inability of the tissue to maintain the high excitation rate imposed by the intramural scroll. This hypothesis is consistent with recent findings of a distinct spatio-temporal organization of electrical activity on the myocardial surface during VF. Specifically, it has been shown that the electrical activity develops distinct domains, each with a spatially uniform dominant frequency. The domains persist for many excitation cycles, from several seconds to several minutes. The frequencies in adjacent domains are usually in simple ratios such as 2:1, 3:2 and 4:3, suggestive of Wenkebach periodicity. Presence of such domains without apparent sustained reentrant activity on the surface is consistent with stable intramural sources of excitation. Demonstration of stable filaments during VF in our transillumination experiments suggests that such sources can be intramural scroll waves.

References

1. Pertsov AM, Jalife J. Scroll Waves in Three-Dimensional Cardiac Muscle. In Zipes DP, Jalife J (eds) **Cardiac Electrophysiology, From Cell to Bedside: Third Edition**, 1999, Chapter 39. WB Saunders Co., Philadelphia, pp 336–344.
2. Berenfeld O, Pertsov AM. Dynamics of intramural scroll waves in a 3-dimensional continuous myocardium with rotational anisotropy. *J Theor Biol* 1999;199:383–394.
3. Wellner M, Berenfeld O, Pertsov AM. Predicting filament drift in twisted anisotropy. *Phys Rev E* 2000;61:1845–1850.
4. Zaitsev AV, Berenfeld O, Mironov SF, et al. Distribution of excitation frequencies on the endocardial and epicardial surfaces of fibrillating ventricular wall. *Circ Res* 2000;86:408–417.
5. Efimov IR, Sidorov V, Cheng Y, et al. Evidence of three-dimensional scroll waves with ribbon-shaped filament as a mechanism of ventricular tachycardia in the isolated rabbit heart. *J Cardiovascular Electrophysiol* 1999;10(11):1452–1462.
6. Vinson M, Mironov S, Mulvey S, et al. Control of spatial orientation and lifetime of scroll rings in excitable media. *Nature* 1997;386:477–480.
7. Baxter WT, Mironov SF, Zaitsev AV, et al. Visualizing excitation waves inside cardiac muscle using transillumination. *Biophys J* 2001;80:516–530.
8. Pertsov AM, Mironov SF, Zaitsev AV, et al. Visualization of stable intramural reentry during fibrillatory activity in perfused sheep right ventricle. *Circulation* 1999;100(18):I-872.

Chapter 9

Action Potential Duration Alternans in a Mono-Cellular Model based on Beeler-Reuter Kinetics

Etienne Pruvot, MD, Vincent Jacquemet, MS,
Jean-Marc Vesin, PhD, Nathalie Virag, PhD,
Olivier Blanc, MS, Jacques Koerfer, MD,
Martin Fromer, MD, Lukas Kappenberger, MD

Introduction

Cardiovascular diseases are the main cause of death in Western countries and account for half a million deaths annually in the USA. Sudden cardiac death (SCD), that results in general from ventricular arrhythmias (VA), accounts for more than 50% of these deaths and its incidence has been estimated as high as 0.1% to 0.2% in the overall population. Shortly after the introduction of the ECG, macroscopic alternans of the T wave (TWA) was recognized as a precursor of VA in various conditions. Recent works have shown that TWA seems to be a harbinger of VA and SCD for structural and electrical diseases. The cellular basis for TWA seems to be located at the membrane level. In experimental conditions[1], but also using computer modeled tissue[2], repolarization alternans in opposite phase between neighboring islands of cardiomyocytes (discordant TWA) fulfilled the requisite conditions for unidirectional block, reentrant propagation and ventricular fibrillation onset. Premature beats (PB) may cause phase resetting during TWA, causing transient reduction in alternans amplitude, but it may also produce a transient TWA in homogeneously repolarized

From Virag N, Blanc O, Kappenberger L (eds): *Computer Simulation and Experimental Assessment of Cardiac Electrophysiology.* ©Futura Publishing Co., Inc., Armonk, NY, 2001.

tissues.[3] Clinical studies have shown that TWA in patients susceptible to VA usually appears for heart rate values above 100 bpm.[4]

From implantable cardioverter defibrillator studies, we know that in the minutes preceding VA onset, ventricular PB increase in frequency, but also that the heart rate does not appear to systematically reach the threshold value for TWA.[5,6] It might be that a properly coupled PB or a sudden increase in heart rate produces a transient TWA, with increased susceptibility to VA after delivery of a second PB. The present study was designed to investigate the role of PB delivery and sudden change in pacing rate on the duration and amplitude of transient alternation of a single cell action potential duration (APD).

Working Hypotheses

We hypothesize that near the first bifurcation in APD, a PB may prolong the duration and amplitude of the transient alternans of a single cell compared to a PB of similar prematurity at a lower pacing rate. In addition, we expect the importance of transient APD alternans triggered by a PB to depend upon the pacing protocol.

Methods

The Beeler-Reuter model[7] used for the present study is meant to simulate a single uncoupled ventricular cell. The membrane kinetics is based on 4 ionic currents (I_{K1}, I_{x1}, I_{Na} and I_s) involving 6 gating variables. The membrane potential evolution $V_m(t)$ is computed from the following equation analogous to the well-known Hodgkin-Huxley formulation:[8]

$$C_m \frac{dV_m}{dt} = I_{K1} + I_{x1} + I_{Na} + I_s - I_{stim} \qquad (1)$$

where C_m is the membrane capacitance and I_{stim} is the excitatory current. I_{stim} will always be a sequence of square impulses of 2 ms duration and 30 $\mu A/cm^2$ intensity (2x diastolic threshold). The system dynamics is described by eight ordinary differential equations, whose numerical integration was performed using a standard approach.[9,10] At rest, the resulting APD has a value of 274 ms.

Two different kinds of stimulation protocols were used in order to investigate both steady state and transient alternans:

1. a protocol with regular pacing rates. Pacing rate is initiated after a first AP of 274 ms. The simulation is run until the steady state is

reached (maximum 300 beats). The last 50 APDs are considered for further analysis;

2. two pacing protocols including a single PB: once steady state APD is achieved, a PB of varying prematurity is delivered. Two PB protocols were defined: the standard protocol (2a) includes a PB followed by a post-extrasystolic pause, while the interpolated protocol (2b) does not include any post-extrasystolic pause.

Suppose that the sequence $\{APD_n\}$ of alternating APDs converges to a well-defined steady state limit APD_{ss}. In this case, the importance of the transient alternans as the result of pacing rate initiation and of the two PB protocols will be quantified as:

$$\sigma = \sqrt{\sum_{n=n_1}^{n_2} (APD_n - APD_{ss})^2} \qquad (2)$$

where the summation begins with the first AP after PB delivery (protocol 2) or with the very first AP (protocol 1) and ends at steady state. The value of σ depends both on the duration and the amplitude of the transient alternans and is similar to the standard deviation, but not normalized. The APD (more precisely APD_{-60} was computed as the time interval the membrane potential remains above a certain threshold, namely –60 mV, corresponding to the excitability threshold.

Results

Regular Pacing Protocol

Figure 1 shows the monotonic concave down restitution curve of the APD as a function of the DI obtained with our single cell Beeler-Reuter model. The point on the curve has a tangent of slope one.

The bifurcation diagram of APDs as a function of regular pacing rates is displayed in Figure 2. For each pacing rate (from 100 bpm to 650 bpm with 1 bpm increment), the last 50 APDs of 300-beat simulations starting from resting potential are measured and displayed on the diagram.

Up to a 216 bpm pacing rate, APDs are stable and do not display a beat-to-beat alternation (1 AP generated for each stimulus). At 216 bpm, the first period doubling is observed, resulting in a stable alternation of short and long APDs. For further increase in pacing rate, only one AP is generated every two stimuli. At higher pacing rates, additional period doublings degenerate towards chaotic dynamics. Between chaotic zones, stability regions are also observed (2 APs for 3 stimuli). The forbidden

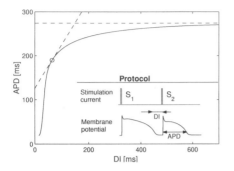

Figure 1. APD_{-60} restitution function for the Beeler-Reuter model. The highlighted point of slope one is related to the bifurcation threshold for stable APD alternans.

bands of APDs are related to the voltage threshold chosen for measuring APDs. As a rule, if the short AP starts within the long AP at a voltage above -60 mV, the short AP is not detected, resulting on the diagram in a single AP of increased duration. This occurs when $APD_{-60} = n$ (BCL, where BCL is the basic cycle length of the pacing rate.

Initiation of regular pacing protocols on the initial APD of 274 ms induces a transient alternation in APDs that converges toward a steady state value. Figure 3 displays σ as a function of the pacing rate up to the bifurcation point leading to stable APD alternans. The transient alternans duration shows a steep increase close to the bifurcation point. More precisely, the curve displays an asymptotic power-law behavior $\sigma \propto |\ BCL - BCL_{bifurc}\ |^{-\lambda}$ for $BCL \rightarrow BCL_{bifurc}$, where $\lambda \approx 0.24$.

Premature Beat Protocols

For each stable pacing rate up to the bifurcation point (216 bpm), the transient alternation in APD between two different pacing protocols (2a and 2b) was compared including a single PB of various prematurities. Protocol 2a included a post-extrasystolic pause, while protocol 2b did not.

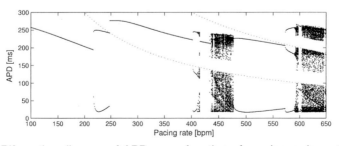

Figure 2. Bifurcation diagram of APDs as a function of regular pacing rates for the Beeler-Reuter model. The last 50 APDs of 300-beat simulations are plotted. The equation for the forbidden bands of APDs (dotted curves) is $APD_{-60} = n \cdot BCL$ for n=1, 2. Note period doublings, chaotic behavior and stability regions for increasing pacing rates.

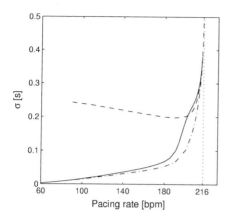

Figure 3. Transient alternans (σ) for the regular pacing protocol (solid curve) as a function of the pacing rate; maximal value of σ over all prematurities computed from the standard protocol (dash-dotted curve) and from the interpolated protocol (dashed curve). The vertical dotted line represents the bifurcation threshold (216 bpm) towards APD period doubling.

Figure 4 (left panel) displays the value of σ as a function of PB prematurity far from the bifurcation point. For the standard protocol, the resulting transient alternans shows a constant σ over the AP, followed by a gradual decrease. For the interpolated protocol, σ increases gradually as PB prematurity decreases, and presents a marked peak at the end of the AP, followed by a steep decrease. Figure 4 (right panel) shows typical sequences of APs starting with a PB of decreasing prematurity. The high σ peak value of the interpolated protocol arises when the PB is of short duration and is followed by an even shorter AP or by a stimulation failure. Note that despite differences in the APs following PB delivery between the

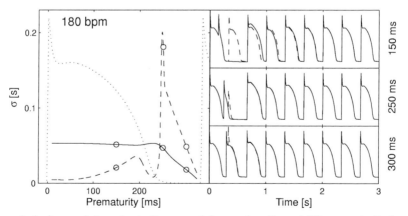

Figure 4. Left panel: transient alternans (σ) as a function of PB prematurity for the standard protocol (solid curve) and for the interpolated protocol (dashed curve) at 180 bpm pacing rate. The steady state action potential (dotted curve) is also superimposed. Right panel: typical examples of APD sequences triggered by PB delivery of decreasing prematurity (150, 250 and 300 ms). Resulting σ values are displayed as circles in the left panel.

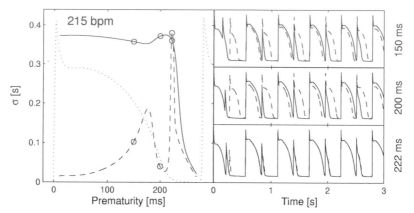

Figure 5. Left panel: transient alternans (σ as a function of PB prematurity for the standard protocol (solid curve) and for the interpolated protocol (dashed curve) at 215 bpm pacing rate. Note that the y-axis scale is twice that of figure 4. The steady state action potential (dotted curve) is also superimposed. Right panel: typical examples of APD sequences triggered by PB delivery of decreasing prematurity (150, 200 and 222 ms). Resulting σ values are displayed as circles in the left panel.

two protocols, the alternation of the APs is of short duration and disappears after 1.5 sec.

Figure 5 displays the value of σ as a function of PB prematurity at 215 bpm, close to the bifurcation point (216 bpm). Roughly, the shape of both curves is similar to figure 4, but σ is clearly increased as compared to lower pacing rate values. Note that the maximum σ value of the standard protocol joins the peak value of the interpolated protocol. In both cases, long DIs following protocol initiation are observed. In the interpolated protocol, the situation becomes similar to the standard protocol, because the first stimulus S_1 fails to generate an AP following PB delivery (222 ms prematurity). In contrast, out of the peak values, σ has a lower value in the interpolated protocol than in the standard one, because the first S_1 in the interpolated protocol reduces the next DI and the resulting transient alternans.

Figure 3 displays the peak value of σ for both PB protocols as a function of pacing rate. Far from the bifurcation point, σ tends to zero except for the interpolated protocol. The main contribution to high σ values for the interpolated protocol is given by the first AP of short duration following PB delivery. Close to bifurcation, σ values display similar asymptotic behaviors for both protocols.

Discussion

The main findings in the present study are that PB delivery and sudden change in pacing rate in a single cell model with steady state APDs produce a transient alternation in APD that increases steeply in amplitude and duration near the pacing rate threshold of the first period doubling.

Period Doubling, Chaotic Behavior and Transient Alternans During Regular Pacing

It has been shown that single cardiac cells based on ionic kinetics models may display nonlinear behavior, period doublings and chaotic dynamics resulting in an alternans of the APD when driven at high pacing rates.[11] APD alternans was reported for restitution curve whose slope was > 1.[2,11] In the present study, our single cell model based on Beeler-Reuter kinetics displayed nonlinear dynamics similar to previous observations.[11] The 216 bpm pacing rate threshold towards stable APD alternans (first bifurcation in Figure 2) corresponds to the point of slope 1 on our restitution curve, and the subsequent period doublings and chaotic dynamics only appear for shorter steady state DIs. Former studies have shown that adjustment of the APD to cycle length shortening is mono-exponential (or linear when plotted against logarithm of cycle[12]). In the present study, the time course of the gradual decrease of APD to changes in pacing rates was assessed in term of transient alternation in APD. The main finding is that abrupt increases in pacing rate produces a transient alternans that increases steeply in amplitude and duration near the first bifurcation, which corresponds to steady state DIs close to the value of slope one. Note that the asymptotic behavior of the transient alternans (Figure 3) as a function of pacing rate follows a power-law. In other words, even though the pacing threshold for stable alternans has not been reached yet, periods of prolonged transient alternans may exist for sudden changes in pacing regimen. Although our findings do not necessarily apply to simulated cardiac tissue or to clinical conditions, it is tempting to extrapolate that sudden increase in heart rate may induce periods of transient TWA, increasing the likelihood of VA in susceptible patients.

Transient Alternans Triggered by PB Delivery

TWA and alternans of APD have been largely involved in the genesis of VA.[1,4,13] Short-coupled PB delivery was shown to experimentally increase dispersion of refractoriness and decrease VF threshold.[14] In tissues displaying discordant alternans, PB delivery or failure to reach one-to-one capture by rapid pacing rates produces considerable increase in the maximum spatial gradient of repolarization, which in turn forms the substrate for unidirectional block and reentry.[2,13] Moreover, PB delivery has been reported to experimentally reverse the phase of mechanoelectrical alternans, but also to elicit a damped form of concordant alternans.[3,4] In our single cell model, short-coupled PB delivery followed by a post-extrasystolic pause produced a nearly constant transient alternans due to failure of the PB to generate an AP. The ensuing time interval added to the post-extrasystolic pause to result in an extremely long DI and APD couple. This was followed by a short DI and APD couple, alternating on an every-other-beat basis towards stable DI and APD values (damped alternans). Transient alternans values progressively decreased once PB delivery started to generate an AP, which in turn decreased the duration of the post-extrasystolic DI. The main finding of our study is that transient alternans increases steeply close to the bifurcation threshold and follows a power-law. In other words, the closer from the stable alternans, the longer and bigger the transient alternans triggered by PB delivery. Although this finding has not been validated in experimental conditions, it may be that spontaneous PB before TWA threshold induce transient alternation in APDs of sufficient duration and amplitude to augment the likelihood of VA onset in susceptible patients.

In alternating tissue, delivery of interpolated PB may prevent or interrupt alternans triggered by initiation of rapid pacing rates.[12] In the present study, the transient alternans triggered by interpolating short coupled PB was always less marked than for PB delivery followed by a post-extrasystolic pause at any pacing rate. In the interpolated protocol, introduction of an additional stimulus S_1 after the PB reduced the following DI and APD, and the damped alternation in APDs. Away from the bifurcation threshold, the interpolated protocol displayed a steep increase in transient alternans for long coupled PB. Failure of the first stimulus S_1 to generate an AP following PB delivery produced a long DI and APD that resulted in an increase in APD alternation, however of very short duration. As a rule, interpolation of a PB in paced single cell model or in experimental conditions reduces the amplitude and duration of the damped APD alternans as compared to PB protocol followed by a post-extrasystolic pause.

References

1. Pastore JM, Girouard SD, Laurita KR, et al. Mechanism linking T-wave alternans to the genesis of cardiac fibrillation. *Circulation* 1999;99(10):1385–1394.
2. Qu Z, Garfinkel A, Chen PS, et al. Mechanisms of discordant alternans and induction of reentry in simulated cardiac tissue. *Circulation* 2000;102(14): 1664–1670.
3. Rubenstein DS, Lipsius SL. Premature beats elicit a phase reversal of mechanoelectrical alternans in cat ventricular myocytes. A possible mechanism for reentrant arrhythmias. *Circulation* 1995;91(1):201–214.
4. Kaufman ES, Mackall JA, Julka B, et al. Influence of heart rate and sympathetic stimulation on arrhythmogenic T wave alternans. *Am J Physiol Heart Circ Physiol* 2000;279(3):H1248–1255.

5. Pruvot E, Thonet G, Vesin JM, et al. Heart rate dynamics at the onset of ventricular tachyarrhythmias as retrieved from implantable cardioverter-defibrillators in patients with coronary artery disease. *Circulation* 2000;101(20): 2398–2404.
6. Vybiral T, Glaeser DH, Goldberger AL, et al. Conventional heart rate variability analysis of ambulatory electrocardiographic recordings fails to predict imminent ventricular fibrillation. *J Am Coll Cardiol* 1993;22(2):557–565.
7. Beeler GW, Reuter H. Reconstruction of the action potential of ventricular myocardial fibres. *J Physiol* 1977;268:177–210.
8. Hodgkin AL, Huxley AF. A quantitative description of membrane current and its application to conduction and excitation in nerve. *J Physiol* 1952;117: 500–544.
9. Rush S, Larsen H. A practical algorithm for solving dynamic membrane equations. *IEEE Trans Biomed Eng* 1978;25(4):389–392.
10. Qu Z, Garfinkel A. An advanced algorithm for solving partial differential equation in cardiac conduction. *IEEE Trans Biomed Eng* 1999;46(9):1166–1168.
11. Vinet A, Chialvo DR, Michaels DC, et al. Nonlinear dynamics of rate-dependent activation in models of single cardiac cells. *Circ Res* 1990;67(6): 1510–1524.
12. Saitoh H, Bailey JC, Surawicz B. Alternans of action potential duration after abrupt shortening of cycle length: Differences between dog Purkinje and ventricular muscle fibers. *Circ Res* 1988;62(5):1027–1040
13. Pastore JM, Rosenbaum DS. Role of structural barriers in the mechanism of alternans-induced reentry. *Circ Res* 2000;87(12):1157–1163.
14. Laurita KR, Girouard SD, Akar FG, et al. Modulated dispersion explains changes in arrhythmia vulnerability during premature stimulation of the heart. *Circulation* 1998;98(24):2774–2780.

Part III.

Mechanical Modeling

Chapter 10

Measurement of Ventricular and Atrial Wall Motion Using Magnetic Resonance with Spin-Tagging

Elliot McVeigh, PhD

Introduction

The measurement of the electrical activity of the heart is a very mature field of research. Intra-cavity electrodes,[1] optical techniques,[2] monophasic action potentials[3] and body surface electrode mapping[4–6] are just some of the methods used to map myocardial electrical activity.

Measuring the local mechanical activity of the heart has been hampered with a lack of nondestructive measurement tools. Implanted beads[7,8] and screws[9] have been used to measure the mechanical activity of the heart in a few isolated regions. Recently, precise and accurate methods for measuring local three-dimensional (3D) myocardial motion with magnetic resonance imaging (MRI) have been developed using presaturation tagging patterns.[10–12] In this article, we will describe the use of these cardiac MRI techniques to produce an image of the local deformation of the heart in the form

[1] Much of the work discussed in this paper was supported through grants from the NHLBI (HL45090, HL45683), the Whitaker Foundation, the Radiological Society of North America, and the American Heart Association. Many of the results and conclusions reported here are from the collaborative efforts of the Cardiac MRI Research Group at Johns Hopkins and the Medical Imaging Group at NHLBI. I would especially like to acknowledge the efforts of Scott Chesnick, Dan Ennis, Frank Evans, Owen Faris, Michael Guttman, Chris Moore, Walter O'Dell, Scott Reeder, Frits Prinzen, Joni Taylor, Brad Wyman, Joshua Tsitlik, Henry Halperin, Bill Hunter and Elias Zerhouni. All of our electrical mapping techniques were taught to us by Bob Lux and Rob McLeod at the CVRTI, University of Utah.

From Virag N, Blanc O, Kappenberger L (eds): *Computer Simulation and Experimental Assessment of Cardiac Electrophysiology.* ©Futura Publishing Co., Inc., Armonk, NY, 2001.

of a myocardial strain image. Using these images we then go on to define the "mechanical activation" of the heart, that is, the time of onset of contraction.

Cardiac Tagging Techniques

Cardiac tagging uses a simple principle: the underlying image is multiplied with a known intensity function and the volume is imaged after some time delay; *the change in shape of the intensity pattern in the image reflects the change in shape of the underlying body containing the intensity pattern.* It was demonstrated by Zerhouni et al. that the simple saturation pulses could be used to create the intensity pattern in MR images.[10] In 1989 Axel and Dougherty proposed a very efficient scheme for generating a large set of parallel planes of saturation throughout the entire imaging volume.[11]

We can break down the process of cardiac tagging into three stages: (1) a saturation pattern is placed in the myocardial tissue with spatially selective radio-frequency pulses, (2) a sequence of MRIs is obtained in which the motion of the saturation pattern can be observed, (3) the motion of the saturation pattern is used to solve for the motion of the myocardium. Figure 1 shows an example of a pair of tagged images of the heart. In this case the saturation pattern is parallel lines.[13]

Analysis of Tagged Images

The objective of the analysis of tagged images is to track the 3D motion of each material point in the heart, and then to compute the six components of the strain tensor at each point. The strain tensor characterizes the *local* deformation of the myocardium, which is a measure of myocardial performance. Bulk translations and rotations of the entire heart may actually dominate the displacement measurements, but these are of limited value as an index of local myocardial contraction. Figure 2 shows a schematic of the process of creating a mapping of strain tensors over the heart from tagged data.

In order to obtain precise quantification of the regional strains, the position of the tags must be measured with a "tag detection" algorithm.[14] Once the relative position of the tags have been determined as a function

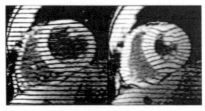

End Diastole   End Systole

Figure 1. An example of tagged MR images of the heart in a normal human volunteer. The tags act as markers which can be tracked with MR imaging for 1/2–1 second.

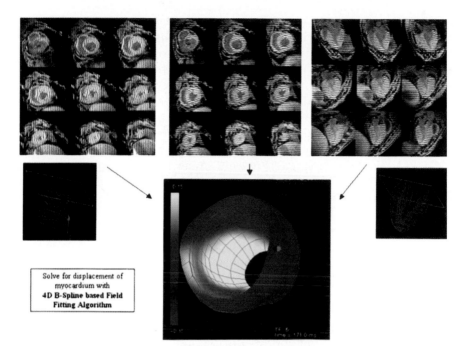

Figure 2. This diagram shows a complete set of tagged images for a single time point in the cardiac cycle. Multiple short axis and long axis planes are sampled at this time point with different acquisitions. These images provide raw displacement data (shown as red wireframes) which is then used to compute the local strains (color-coded in the model view).

of time, these data can be used to estimate the strain tensor at each point in the myocardium. One method for doing this is a displacement field model based on B-splines.[15]

Analysis of Myocardial Function During Asynchronous Activation

In order to evaluate the relationship between electrical excitation and the onset of mechanical contraction, MR tagging experiments were performed during ectopic pacing in anesthetized normal dogs.[16,17] When systolic contraction was evoked by right atrial pacing, the left ventricle (LV) was excited via the normal pathway of the Purkinje system and the pattern of mechanical activation was found to be very uniform as a function of position. However, when the heart was paced from a ventricular site, significant asynchronous and spatially heterogeneous contraction was observed.

The precise sequence of events during ectopic excitation was particularly evident on the color encoded strain images. Figure 3 shows the evolution in time of the circumferential component of the 3D strain tensor (E_{cc}) evaluated at the mid-wall for the three pacing sites; this component of the strain tensor closely matches muscle fiber shortening at the mid-wall of the LV. For atrial pacing (normal activation pathway) muscle shortening evolves relatively homogeneously over the ventricle; this is shown as the uniformly increasing blue color over the ventricle in the top row of Figure 3. With ventricular pacing, a clear focus of early mechanical shortening was observed at the pacing site, followed by propagation of a contraction wavefront to the opposite side of the heart. This is seen as the blue "wave" of muscle shortening emanating from the LV freewall pacing site (10 o'clock) in the middle row of Fig. 3 and from the RV apex site (5 o'clock) in the bottom row of Figure 3. A second interesting observation was the significant "prestretch" of the late activated myocardium remote from the pacing site, shown as a bright yellow color. This prestretch was quite pronounced (15%–20%) and occurred in the first 100 ms after the ventricular pacing pulse.

An alternative way of visualizing the contraction pattern is to graph the time course of strain for each material point of the LV. Each graph can be mapped to a position in an array that corresponds to a position in the LV. An example of such an *LV strain map* is shown in Figure 4 where the sequence of mechanical shortening (mid-wall E_{cc}) for the left ventricular base and right ventricular apex pacing sites are plotted. The LV strain maps are an excellent method for observing the rapid rate of prestretch in

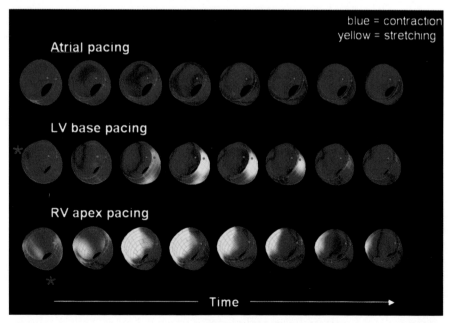

Figure 3. Dynamic local strain images of the paced heart. The blue color represents muscle shortening in the circumferencial direction, yellow represents stretching of that muscle.

Left Ventricular Strain Map: Circumferential Shortening

* RV apex pacing, * LV base pacing

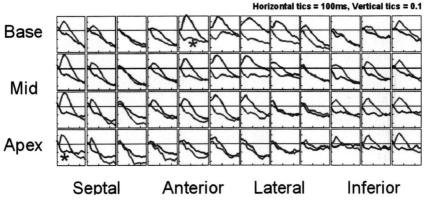

Figure 4. An array of graphs showing the local values for circumferencial shortening (or stretching) during pacing. Each box represents approximately 1/2 cc of tissue. The horizontal axis represents time, the vertical axis represents strain. Detailed analysis is given in the text.

the passive, late activated regions (see columns 1–2, and 11–12 for LV base pacing, columns 4–8 for right ventricle [RV] apex pacing) and the rapid contraction at the pacing site (columns 4–6 for LV base pacing, columns 1,2,12 for RV apex pacing). Also demonstrated directly from these plots is the increased "stroke" or total dynamic range of the strain in the pre-stretched region. Because the majority of this shortening occurs during the ejection phase (with high ventricular pressure), the prestretched region is performing increased contractile work.[18]

While asynchronous mechanical activation was obvious from both the color encoded strain images shown in Figure 3 and the LV strain map showing E_{cc} versus time, we can also define the "mechanical activation time" as the time at which the muscle begins to shorten. This will correspond to the time at which the prestretch or ventricular filling reaches a peak, as shown in the LV strain maps of Figure 4. For those curves in Figure 4 that have an easily detectable maximum in the prestretch of the tissue, this definition works well.

The mechanical data described above can be obtained from a dog in vivo while simultaneously measuring epicardial electrical excitation maps with a sock electrode array placed around the heart. From these data, maps of both mechanical activation (time of onset of shortening) and electrical activation (time of maximum negative slope in unipolar recordings) were computed. Color encoded activation maps are shown in Figure 5, showing the high degree of correlation between the electrical activation

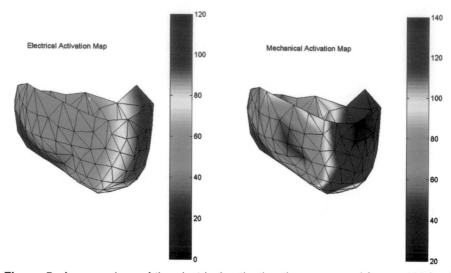

Figure 5. A comparison of the electrical activation time measured from a 128-lead electrode sock, and the "mechanical activation time" computed from the local myocardial shortening over the LV and RV in a dog heart. These initial results show promise for a method of mapping activation through noninvasive mechanical mapping.

map and the mechanical activation map, as it is defined here. This is not surprising in the normal heart; the change in this dependence in pathology, such as regional ischemia, and during administration of drugs that affect E-C coupling is just now under investigation.

Discussion

Strain imaging with MRI tagging now gives us a new tool for studying the temporal kinetics of myocardial contraction. Because this technique is non-invasive, it can be applied in patients with no risk. Under conditions where the heart is beating in a reproducible manner, high resolution mechanical activation maps can be achieved, and these will correlate with the underlying electrical activation. The strain imaging data could possibly be used as a further boundary condition with torso ECG data to perform more accurate reconstruction of epicardial electrophysiological maps from body surface potentials.[4] One direction of research that is now possible is the study of the effect of mechanical stretch on the electrical nature of the heart. It has been demonstrated that rapid prestretch will stimulate depolarization of the myocardium especially in regions that have the greatest compliance and experience greater relative stretch,[3] and that the timing of the application of prestretch determines if an arrhythmic depolarization of the LV will occur.[19] This new strain imaging technique combined with simultaneous electrical mapping will allow us to investigate the local prestretch needed to generate these arrhythmic beats.

References

1. Liu ZW, Jia P, Biblo LA, et al. Endocardial potential mapping from a noncontact nonexpandable catheter: A feasibility study. *Ann Biomed Eng* 1998; 26:994–1009.
2. Salama G. Optical measurement of transmembrane potential. In Loew L (ed). **Spectroscopic Membrane Probes Vol. III**, Boca Raton, CRC, 1988, pp. 137–199.
3. Franz MR, Cima R, Wang D, et al. Electrophysiological effects of myocardial stretch and mechanical determinants of stretch-activated arrhythmias. *Circulation* 1992;86: 968–978.
4. MacLeod RS, Brooks DH. Recent progress in inverse problems in electrocardiology. *IEEE Eng Med Biol Mag* 1998;17:73–83.
5. Burnes JE, Taccardi B, Rudy Y. A noninvasive imaging modality for cardiac arrhythmias. *Circulation* 2000;102:2152–2158.
6. Brooks DH, MacLeod RS. Electrical Imaging of the Heart. *IEEE Signal Processing Magazine* 1997;14:24–42.
7. Waldman LK, Fung YC, Covell JW. Transmural myocardial deformation in the canine left ventricle. *Circ Res* 1985;57:152–163.
8. Douglas AS, Rodriguez EK, O'Dell W, et al. Unique strain history during ejection in canine left ventricle. *Am J Physiol* 1991;260:H1596–H1611.
9. Hansen DE, Daughters GT, Alderman EL, et al. Effect of volume loading, pressure loading, and inotropic stimulation on left ventricular torsion in humans. *Circulation* 1991;83:1315–1326.
10. Zerhouni EA, Parish DM, Rogers WJ, et al. Human heart: Tagging with MR imaging-a method for noninvasive assessment of myocardial motion. *Radiology* 1988;169:59–63.
11. Axel L, Dougherty L. MR imaging of motion with spatial modulation of magnetization. *Radiology* 1989;171:841–845.
12. McVeigh ER. MRI of myocardial function: Motion tracking techniques. *Magn Reson Imag* 1996;14:137–150.
13. McVeigh ER, Atalar E. Cardiac tagging with breath-hold cine MRI. *Magn Reson Med* 1992;28:318–327.
14. Guttman MA, Prince JL, McVeigh ER. Tag and contour detection in tagged MR images of the left ventricle. *IEEE Trans Med Imag* 1994;13:74–88.
15. Ozturk C, McVeigh ER. Four-dimensional B-spline based motion analysis of tagged MR images: Introduction and in vivo validation. *Phys Med Biol* 2000;45:1683–1702.
16. McVeigh ER, Prinzen FW, Wyman BT, et al. Imaging asynchronous mechanical activation of the paced heart with tagged MRI. *Magn Reson Med* 1998;39:507–513.
17. Wyman BT, Hunter WC, Prinzen FW, et al. Mapping propagation of mechanical activation in the paced heart with MRI tagging. *Am J Physiol* 1999; 276:H881–H891.

18. Prinzen FW, Hunter WC, Wyman BT, et al. Mapping of regional myocardial strain and work during ventricular pacing: Experimental study using magnetic resonance imaging tagging. *J Am Coll Cardiol* 1999;33:1735–1742.
19. Zabel M, Koller BS, Sachs F, et al. Stretch-induced voltage changes in the isolated beating heart: Importance of the timing of stretch and implications for stretch-activated ion channels. *Cardiovasc Res* 1996;32:120–130.

Chapter 11

Computational and Experimental Modeling of Ventricular Electromechanical Interactions

Andrew McCulloch, PhD, Derrick Sung, MS, Mary Ellen Thomas, MS, Anushka Michailova, MS

Introduction

Perturbations in ventricular mechanical loading can be arrhythmogenic and have been associated with sudden cardiac death in patients suffering from congestive heart failure, dilated cardiomyopathy, or ventricular volume overload.[1–3] Stretch-induced changes in action potential propagation or repolarization could provide a mechanism for mechanically induced arrhythmias. However, there is a paucity of information regarding the effects of altered load on conduction velocity. The few existing reports present an unclear picture; some of the discrepancies may be due to the varying techniques used.

Stretch activated channels (SACs) have been identified as a potential cellular mechanism for mechanoelectric feedback.[4] Mechano-sensitive ion channels have been identified in the ventricular myocardium of several species, both nonspecific cation or K^+ specific channels.[5–7] The aminoglycoside antibiotic streptomycin has been reported to block stretch activated channels.[8]

Past studies of cardiac mechanoelectric feedback have all used contact electrodes to measure the electrical activity of the heart. The required

[1] This research was supported in part by NSF grant BES-9634974 and the National Biomedical Computation Resource, NIH P41 grant RR08605. Derrick Sung was supported by NIH training grant T32HL07444. Mary Ellen Thomas was a NSF scholar.

From Virag N, Blanc O, Kappenberger L (eds): *Computer Simulation and Experimental Assessment of Cardiac Electrophysiology.* ©Futura Publishing Co., Inc., Armonk, NY, 2001.

physical contact between the measuring device and the myocardium leaves the measurements open to the possibility of mechanically induced electrical artifact.[9] Optical mapping provides a noncontact means of measuring cardiac electrical activity through the use of a voltage-sensitive fluorescent dye. The spatial resolution from this technique is higher than that of conventional electrode arrays and is thus particularly desirable for conduction velocity measurements. In the present study, we used optical mapping to investigate the effects of increased left ventricular loading on apparent epicardial conduction velocity and action potential duration. Streptomycin was used to assess if any of the observed electrophysiological changes might be governed by stretch activated channels. A preliminary report of this study has been submitted to the 2001 ASME Summer Bioengineering meeting.

Methods

Experiments were conducted in 11 isolated Langendorff-perfused rabbit hearts. A balloon in the left ventricle was connected to a fluid-filled pressure transducer and a volume infusion pump. Following aortic cannulation, hearts were perfused with Tyrode's solution and allowed to actively contract. The initial volume in the balloon was adjusted to achieve an end diastolic pressure (EDP) of $\approx$0 mmHg. The myocardium was preconditioned three times by infusing and withdrawing volume into the balloon at a rate of 10 mL/min to a peak EDP of 30 mmHg. On the final preconditioning run, the volume at EDP = 30 mmHg was recorded, and the LV was loaded to this set volume (V1) during the subsequent loading protocols throughout the experiment. 10.4 μM of the voltage-sensitive dye, DI-4-ANEPPS dissolved in DMSO was injected in a 10-mL bolus of Tyrode's solution into the coronary arteries via the aortic cannula. Prior to the acquisition of optical measurements, the electromechanical uncoupling agent 2,3 butanedione monoxime (BDM, 12.5 mM) was also added to the perfusate to prevent motion artifact. BDM was washed out immediately after each data acquisition was completed. The heart was paced at twice diastolic threshold (cycle length = 300 msec) from the left ventricular epicardium near the apex. In 5 of the 11 hearts, the above loading protocol was repeated after the perfusate was switched to one containing 200 μM streptomycin. The heart was allowed to stabilize for 15 minutes before each cycle of loading and data acquisition was repeated.

The hardware configuration for optical mapping has been described previously.[10] Fluorescence images of the LV free wall (lateral view) were captured with a digital CCD camera (Dalsa, Waterloo, Ontario) at a speed of 399 frames per second and a resolution of 128 × 128 pixels. The image processing and analysis of the optical data has been detailed elsewhere.[10,11] After the signals were filtered, key features from the optical action potentials were extracted and mapped. Activation times were identified as the time at the maximum first derivative $(dF/dt)max$ of the optical action potential upstroke. To calculate action potential repolarization, the peak signal following the upstroke was identified. Time of repolarization was computed by determining the time at which the optical action potential had recovered 20% and 80% from its peak value. The difference between the repolarization and activation times was taken to be the action potential duration (APD).

The gross geometry of each heart was reconstructed from orthogonal biplane images of the lateral and posterior views, and a finite-element surface was then fitted to the boundary data yielding a three-dimensional surface model of the epicardium. The activation times, maximum derivatives of the upstroke, and APD times were then mapped on to the surface of the finite element model and fit by linear least squares as a scalar field variable. The resulting model allowed the electrophysiological variables to be expressed as functions of the three-dimensional coordinates of the epicardial geometry. Conduction velocities and APD were compared using a repeated measures analysis of variance (ANOVA) with distance from the pacing site as the within factor and loading state and streptomycin interventions as between factors.

Results

Pacing was initiated near the apex of the left ventricle so that the longest path of propagation could be analyzed (Figure 1). Total mean apparent conduction velocity averaged over all distances decreased from 398 ± 37 mm/sec in the unloaded pre-control state to 288 ± 16 mm/sec in the loaded state (p = 0.028). By ANOVA, the interaction effect between load state and distance from pacing site was not significant (p = 0.26), suggest-

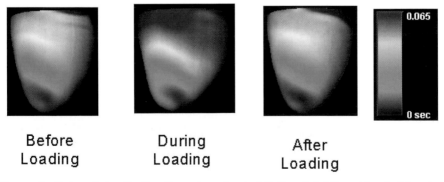

| Before | During | After |
| Loading | Loading | Loading |

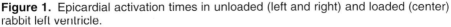

Figure 1. Epicardial activation times in unloaded (left and right) and loaded (center) rabbit left ventricle.

ing that the decrease in conduction velocity in response to ventricular load was not changed at the different locations on the surface of the heart. There was no significant change in apparent conduction velocity between the two unloaded states ($p = 0.96$). $(dF/dt)max$ of the optical action potential upstroke decreased about 5%, but a decrease of this amount or greater would be expected simply as a result of slowed conduction, so decreased membrane excitability is unlikely to explain the observed stretch-dependent slowing. Adding streptomycin to the perfusate did not change the overall conduction velocities ($p > 0.43$) or the response of apparent conduction velocity to load ($p = 0.40$), suggesting that SACs are unlikely to play a primary role in this effect. There was no significant difference in the relative decrease in apparent conduction velocity with respect to distance from the pacing site, indicating that the effect is present transmurally throughout the myocardium.

Total mean APD_{20} increased from an unloaded precontrol value of 0.103 ± 0.004 seconds to 0.116 ± 0.004 seconds when load was applied ($p = 0.006$). Following removal of the load, APD_{20} recovered to a value of 0.110 ± 0.003 seconds which was not statistically significant from the unloaded precontrol state ($p = 0.21$). Total mean APD_{80} increased from an unloaded precontrol value of 0.181 ± 0.004 seconds to 0.209 ± 0.004 seconds following the application of ventricular load ($p < 0.0001$). APD_{80} recovered to 0.194 ± 0.004 seconds in the unloaded postcontrol state, which was still significantly higher than the precontrol value ($p = 0.0003$) suggesting that there may be a longer time course involved with recovery of APD_{80} following load. Streptomycin did not affect the response of APD_{20} ($p = 0.58$) or APD_{80} ($p = 0.95$) to changes in ventricular loading states. Streptomycin also did not have a significant effect on overall APD at either the 20% ($p = 0.59$) or 80% ($p = 0.36$) repolarization levels.

Model Analysis

We investigated the possibility that altered intracellular calcium cycling via length-dependent activation may contribute to the increase in APD with stretch. Using a modification by Michailova and McCulloch[12] (Figure 2) of the canine ionic model by Winslow et al.,[13] we simulated the effects of stretch by increasing the on-rate for calcium binding to troponin and studied the influence on APD. This preliminary analysis showed that under some circumstances the resulting decrease in free myoplasmic calcium during systole was able to prolong relaxation somewhat (Figure 3).

Discussion

We have shown that acute loading of the left ventricle decreases apparent epicardial conduction velocity and increases APD in the isolated

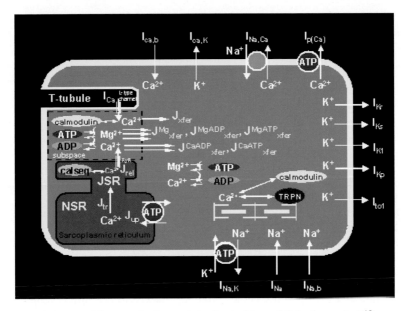

Figure 2. Myocyte ionic model adapted from Michailova et al.[12]

rabbit heart, and these responses do not appear to be mediated by a stretch-activated current. The decrease in conduction velocity could have potential arrhythmogenic consequences by decreasing the wavelength for reentry. In this way, mechanoelectric could contribute to arrhythmias associated with altered ventricular loading conditions. We also observed a

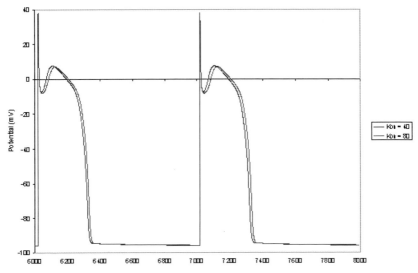

Figure 3. Increasing troponin affinity for calcium prolonged the action potential in a preliminary model.

prolongation of action potential duration with loading that was not blocked by streptomycin. A model analysis suggests that altered intracellular calcium cycling could be a contributing mechanism.

References

1. Reiter MJ. Effects of mechano-electrical feedback: Potential arrhythmogenic influence in patients with congestive heart failure. *Cardiovasc Res* 1996;32 (1):44–51.
2. Huang SK, Messer JV, Denes P. Significance of ventricular tachycardia in idiopathic dilated cardiomyopathy: Observations in 35 patients. *Am J Cardiol* 1983;51(3):507–512.
3. Dean JW, Lab MJ. Arrhythmia in heart failure: Role of mechanically induced changes in electrophysiology. *Lancet* 1989;1(8650):1309–1312.
4. Hu H, Sachs F. Stretch-activated ion channels in the heart. *J Mol Cell Cardiol* 1997;29(6):511–523.
5. Ruknudin A, Sachs F, Bustamante JO. Stretch-activated ion channels in tissue-cultured chick heart. *Am J Physiol* 1993;264(Pt 2):H960–H972.
6. Craelius W, Chen V, El-Sherif N. Stretch activated ion channels in ventricular myocytes. *Biosci Rep* 1988;8(5):407–414.
7. Sigurdson WS, et al. Stretch activation of a K+ channel in molluscan heart cells. *J Exp Biol* 1987;127:191–209.
8. Salmon AH, et al. Effect of streptomycin on wall-stress-induced arrhythmias in the working rat heart. *Cardiovasc Res* 1997;34(3):493–503.
9. Lab MJ. Mechanoelectric feedback (transduction) in heart: Concepts and implications. *Cardiovasc Res* 1996;32(1):3–14.
10. Sung D, Omens JH, McCulloch AD. Model-based analysis of optically mapped epicardial activation patterns and conduction velocity. *Ann Biomed Eng* 2000;28(9):1085–1092.
11. Sung D, et al. Phase-shifting prior to spatial filtering enhances optical recordings of cardiac action potential propagation. *Ann Biomed Eng* 2001. Submitted.
12. Michailova A, McCulloch AD, Modeling Ca^{2+} transients and Ca^{2+} and Mg^{2+} exchange with ATP and ADP during excitation-contraction coupling in ventricular myocytes. *Biophys J* 2001. Submitted.
13. Winslow RL, et al. Mechanisms of altered excitation-contraction coupling in canine tachycardia-induced heart failure, II: Model studies. *Circ Res* 1999;84(5):571–586.

Part IV.

Towards Whole Heart Modeling

Chapter 12

Simulation of Cardiac Electrophysiology and Electrocardiography

Frank B. Sachse, PhD, Christian Werner, MS, Gunnar Seeman, MS

Introduction

Knowledge concerning the development and propagation of the electrical excitation in the myocardium as well as the resulting electrical fields is of importance for the understanding of the physiological and pathophysiological behavior of the heart. The standard approachs to achieve this knowledge are measurements with invasive and noninvasive methods, i.e., electrocardiography and magnetocardiography.

This chapter illustrates an approach by computer aided simulation based on different types of models and numerical methods to calculate electric fields. Conductivity models were derived from a realistically shaped, highly detailed anatomical model. Cardiac source models were obtained by a model of the excitation propagation within the heart. The numerical methods were used to solve the forward problem, which consists of calculating the electrical field distribution arising from sources.

The intention of the presented approach is to provide simulation results with relatively low demands on computing resources. Nonetheless, the simulations have to be accurate enough to obtain realistically shaped electrocardiograms for physiologic and pathophysiologic cases.

From Virag N, Blanc O, Kappenberger L (eds): *Computer Simulation and Experimental Assessment of Cardiac Electrophysiology.* ©Futura Publishing Co., Inc., Armonk, NY, 2001.

Anatomical and Conductivity Models

The anatomical model, that forms the foundation of this study, results from the MEET Man project (Models for Simulation of Electromagnetic, Elastomechanic and Thermal Behavior of Man).[1] The purpose of this project is the creation of models for simulating the physical behavior of man.

The model originates from computer tomographic scans and thin-section photos of the Visible Man dataset,[2] which is provided by the National Library of Medicine, Bethesda, Maryland (USA). The image data resulted

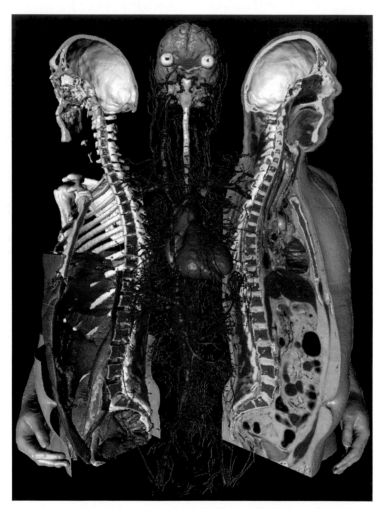

Figure 1. Upper part of anatomical model. Surfaces of different tissue types are visualized.

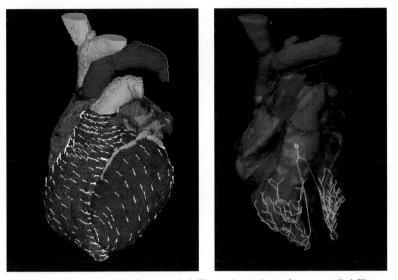

Figure 2. Anatomical model of heart. (a) The orientation of myocardial fibers at the ventricular surface is indicated by white lines. (b) Specialized cardiac conduction system in anatomical context. The yellow lines show the locations of fibers. The surface of the myocardium is visualized semi-transparent.

from applying different techniques of medical imaging to the body of a 39-year-old, 1.8 m tall male weighing 93 kg, who was sentenced to death. The model was created using advanced strategies of digital image processing.[3,4]

The anatomical model (Figure 1) is stored in a three-dimensional dataset, which consists of approximately 400 millions cubic voxels. Each voxel has a size of 1 mm $\times$ 1 mm $\times$ 1 mm and is assigned to one out of forty different tissue classes. The model includes the orientation of muscle fibers. Therefore, an additional orientation dataset is used. Two angles, $\phi \in [0...\pi]$ and $\theta \in [0...\pi]$, were assigned to every voxel that belongs to the tissue classes skeletal or cardiac muscle (Figure 2).

A further model was integrated in the anatomical model describing parts of the excitation conduction system, which needs a relatively high spatial resolution. The conduction system is created semi-automatically, because limitations of the image data regarding resolution and contrast made it impossible to create the conduction system automatically by means of digital image processing. The conduction system is represented by a tree composed of nodes and edges (Figure 2).

The anatomical model was used to derive anatomical models with lower resolution by determining the occurrence of tissue class in every single voxel. The most frequently occurring tissue class was assigned to each voxel in the reduced model.

Conductivity models were derived from these anatomical models by assigning an electrical conductivity to each tissue class. These partly anisotropic, frequency dependent electrical conductivities were taken from in vitro measurement.[5,6] The conductivity is represented by a second-order symmetric tensor.

Numerical Methods

Different tasks in electrophysiology can be solved using the generalized Poisson's equation for electrical conduction:

$$\nabla(\sigma^\beta \nabla \phi) + f = 0 \tag{1}$$

where ϕ represents the potential, σ^β the second-order symmetric conductivity tensor and the current density source. Poisson's equation has to be fulfilled at every point in the spatial domain. Different methods allow the numerical solution of Poisson's equation, e.g. the finite differences and finite element method.

Using the finite differences method in conjunction with an appropriate spatial pointwise discretization allows Poisson's equation to be directly transformed to a system of linear equations. The dimension of this system is determined by the number of discretization points. The finite element method can be applied after conversion of Poisson's equation to an integral over the volume V, e.g., with the method of Galerkin:[7]

$$I = \iiint_V \frac{1}{2}(\nabla \phi)^T (\sigma^\beta \nabla \phi) + f \ \phi \ dx \ dy \ dz \tag{2}$$

Also, the application of the finite element method needs an appropriate spatial discretization and delivers a system of linear equations with a dimension determined by the number of discretization points. The system is modified to include boundary conditions, which describe the potential and its gradient in given regions.

In this study the finite difference method was chosen to solve the forward problem. The solution of the linear system was determined using an iterative solver based on the Full Multigrid Algorithm.[8] An appropriate initial solution for the iterative solving was chosen to accelerate the calculations, e.g., a significant decrease of calculations can be found for simulation of complete heart cycles.

Models of Excitation Propagation

Different approaches for the macroscopic excitation propagation were developed in the past few years:

- Cellular automatons. Rules are included defining the time delay and the neighborhood for the propagation.[9,10]
- Excitable dynamics equations or reaction diffusion systems.[11,12]
- Resistor networks/monodomain models in conjunction with electrophysiologic cell models. These models incorporate the effect of coupling the intracellular space with gap junctions.[13,14]
- Bidomain models. Bidomain models are an extension of monodomain models including the effects of the extracellular space.[15,16]

Some of these models cannot cope with a simulation of the whole heart because even high performance computer systems cannot presently deliver enough computation velocity and memory. Therefore, a computationally efficient cellular automaton is used in this work.[10] The automaton is based on the anatomical model and takes into account tissue and fiber orientation specific variations of the excitation velocity as well as the stimulus dependent variations of the transmembrane potential. The parametrisation of the automaton was derived by simulations with bidomain models of excitation propagation.

Cardiac Sources

A cardiac source model was applied to determine the current density source,[17,10] which is needed to compute the electrical potential distribution in the body. The model bases on a bidomain description of the tissue distribution in the heart and takes into account the potential across the cell membrane delivered by the model of excitation propagation. Further, the model takes into account tissue specific extra- and intracellular conductivities as well as specific boundary conditions, e.g., at the borders of via gap junctions coupled regions of myocardium. The calculated sources are described by the impressed current per volume unit for each voxel of the model.

Results and Conclusions

This work describes methods to simulate the cardiac electrophysiology and the electrocardiography. Outcomes of the simulation of physio-

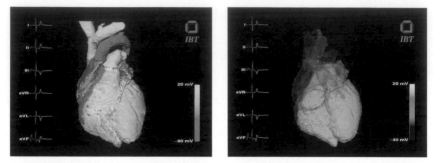

Figure 3. Simulation of sinus rhythm. The images show the transmembrane potential distribution in a (left) surface and (right) volume based representation.

logic excitation propagation are demonstrated in Figure 3. The resulting potential distributions and electrocardiographies are illustrated in Figure 4. Outcomes of the simulation of a pathology of the excitation propagation are demonstrated in Figure 5.

The presented methods can be applied to gain knowledge concerning the cardiac electrophysiology and pathophysiology as well as the electrocardiography, e.g., for diagnosis and educational purposes in electrocardiology.

The development of the simulation system showed that the selection of appropriate models is a task of great importance. This selection can be supported by analysis and comparison of solutions obtained from numerical calculations based on a set of exemplary models. In this way different properties of models, i.e., inhomogeneities and anisotropy of tissue, spatial resolution of models and their influence on solutions have been examined in previous studies.[18,19]

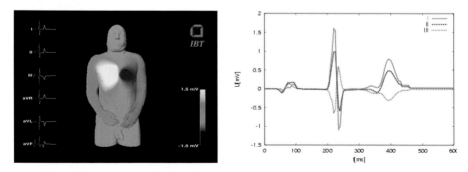

Figure 4. Simulation of sinus rhythm. The images show (left) the body surface potential distribution and (right) standard leads of electrocardiography.

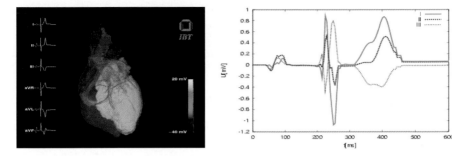

Figure 5. Simulation of a right bundle branch block. The images show (left) the trans-membrane potential distribution and (right) the resulting electrocardiogram.

References

1. Institut für Biomedizinische Technik, Universität Karlsruhe, Germany. MEET Man project. www-ibt.etec.uni-karlsruhe.de/MEETMan.
2. Ackerman MJ. Viewpoint: The Visible Human Project. *J Biocommunication* 1991;18:14.
3. Sachse FB, Werner CD, Müller M, et al. Preprocessing of the Visible Man dataset for the generation of macroscopic anatomical models. *Proc. First Users Conference of the National Library of Medicine's Visible Human Project* 1996.
4. Sachse FB, Wolf M, Werner CD, et al. Extension of anatomical models of the human body: Three dimensional interpolation of muscle fiber orientation based on restrictions. *J of Computing and Information Technology* 1998; 6(1):95–101.
5. Gabriel S, Lau RW, Gabriel C. The dielelectric properties of biological tissues: II. Measurements in the frequency range 10 Hz to 20 GHz. *Phys Med Biol* 1996;41:2251–2269.
6. Gabriel S, Lau RW, Gabriel C. The dielelectric properties of biological tissues: III. Parametric models for the dielectric spectrum of tissues. *Phys Med Biol* 1996;41:2271–2293.
7. Schwarz HR. **Methode der finiten Elemente**.Stuttgart, Teubner, 3rd edition, 1991.
8. Press WH, Teukolsky SA, Vetterling WT, et al. **Numerical Recipes in C**. Cambridge University Press, 2nd edition, Cambridge, New York, Melbourne, 1992.
9. Eifler WJ, Plonsey R. A cellular model for the simulation of activation in the ventricular myocardium. *J Electrocardiol* 1975;8,(2):117–128.
10. Werner CD, Sachse FB, Dössel O. Electrical excitation propagation in the human heart. CardioModel 2000, Computer Models of the Heart: Theory and Clinical Application 2000;2:2. *Int J of Bioelectromagnetism* 2000; ISSN:1456–7865.
11. FitzHugh RA. Impulses and physiological states in theoretical models of nerve membrane. *Biophys J* 1961;1:445–466.

12. Rogers JM, McCulloch AD. A collocation-Galerkin finite element model of cardiac action potential propagation. *IEEE Trans on Biomed Eng* 1994;41: 743–757.
13. Rudy Y, Quan W. Mathematical model of reentry of cardiac excitation. *Proc Computers in Cardiology* 1989;16:135–136.
14. Virag N, Blanc O, Vesin J-M, et al. Study of the mechanisms of arrhythmias in an anatomical computer model of human atria. *Proc Computers in Cardiology* 1999;26:113–116.
15. Henriquez CS, Plonsey R. A bidomain model for simulating propagation in multicellular cardiac tissue. *Proc of the Annual International Conference of the IEEE Engineering in Medicine and Biology Society* 1989;(4):1266.
16. Sepulveda NG, Wikswo JP. Bipolar stimulation of cardiac tissue using an anisotropic bidomain model. *J Cardiovasc Electrophysiol* 1994;5:258–267.
17. Werner CD, Sachse FB, Dössel O. Applications of the visible man dataset in electrocardiology: Simulation of the electrical excitation propagation. *Proc Second Users Conference of the National Library of Medicine's Visible Human Project* 1998:69–79.
18. Klepfer RN, Johnson CR, MacLeod RS. The effects of inhomogeneities and anisotropies on electrocardiographic fields: A 3-D finite-element study. *IEEE Trans on Biomed Eng* 1997;44:706–719.
19. Sachse FB, Werner CD, Meyer-Waarden K, et al. Comparison of solutions to the forward problem in electrophysiology with homogeneous, heterogeneous and anisotropic impedance models. *Biomedizinische Technik* 1997;42 1:277–280.

Chapter 13

Modeling of Arbitrary 3D Geometries:
Application to the Atria and Ventricles
David M. Harrild, PhD, Craig S. Henriquez, PhD

Introduction

One of the long-term objectives in modeling the heart has been to integrate membrane-level description of ion-fluxes into anatomically realistic, three-dimensional representations of the tissue structure. To accomplish this, a procedure must be used that represents the complex anatomy with a computational mesh, allows the assignment of material and membrane properties to that mesh, uses a numerical method and algorithm for tractable simulation, and creates various output that can be subsequently analyzed. In this chapter, we describe the approach we used to create a realistic three-dimensional model of the human atria and demonstrate that large-scale simulation of cardiac dynamics is possible using algorithms developed for distributed parallel computers.

Methods

Mesh Construction

The process begins by first representing the anatomy with a set of stereolithography (STL) triangulated surfaces of the heart obtained from

[1] This work was supported by a grant of supercomputer time from the North Carolina Supercomputing Center, NIH/NIGMS Medical Scientist Training Program Grant GM-07171, NSF Grant DBI 9974533, and NIH Grant R29-HL57473.

From Virag N, Blanc O, Kappenberger L (eds): *Computer Simulation and Experimental Assessment of Cardiac Electrophysiology.* ©Futura Publishing Co., Inc., Armonk, NY, 2001.

Viewpoint Digital (Islandia, NY). These surfaces were subsequently modified to give more realistic dimensions of the anatomic substructures.

Once the anatomical surfaces are obtained, the next step is to use them to produce a multiblock mesh. As the name implies, a multiblock (or "block structured") mesh is comprised of a set of subblocks. Each of these blocks is structured, that is, characterized by a row-by-column-by-layer organization. The multiblock mesh begins as a cube centered on the anatomy of interest. Subblocks are removed from the cube until only the remaining blocks capture the essential features of the anatomy, grossly. The faces of adjacent blocks are merged to form rounded surfaces and the mesh faces are projected to the anatomical surfaces (see Figure 1). In this way, the mesh comes to resemble the object of interest. The mesh building process is accomplished using the software product TrueGrid (XYZ Scientific Applications, Inc., Livermore, CA).

The multiblock mesh describes the geometry of the anatomical configuration. To represent both the tissue and its architecture, a fiber direction must be assigned throughout the mesh, and the tissue conductivity must be defined everywhere. The fiber direction itself can come from careful histological examination of the tissue or through diffusion tensor magnetic resonance imaging (MRI). In this model, the assignment process takes advantage of the multiblock nature of the mesh. Because the blocks are defined such that they represent specific anatomic structures, and conform to tissue areas with specific properties, the properties are assigned within each region separately.

Assignment of Tissue Properties

The mesh is used with the fiber direction and conductivity information to produce a matrix. The coefficients of the matrix are provided by a three-dimensional variation of a Finite Volume method that operates on hexahedral elements.[1] The matrix incorporates all of the information regarding interelement electrical connectivity and serves to govern the diffusive spread of current within the mesh. Whenever two elements are electrically connected, a change in the potential of one will influence the potential at the other. This reality is reflected by the presence of a nonzero coefficient in the matrix at the row of the first unknown and column of the second (and visa-versa, due to the mesh symmetry and current conservation). In practice, a sparse matrix format is used to save disk storage space. The format used in our case requires the storage of only the nonzero coefficients in the matrix and their positions. Seventy-five megabytes of storage space are required for a matrix incorporating 243,080 elements.[2]

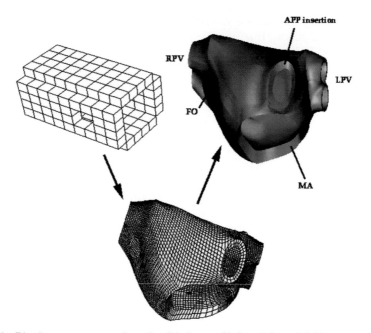

Figure 1. Block structure, mesh and solid views of left atrial model. Named structures are: left atrial appendage (APP); right and left pulmonary veins (RPV and LPV); mitral annulus (MA) and fossa ovalis (FO). The full model uses 8 such blocks.

Algorithms for Efficient Simulation

The matrix is usually initially characterized by a large bandwidth. The bandwidth is defined as the greatest displacement of any non-zero element from the diagonal, for any row, divided by the matrix size. The custom program used to simulate the propagation of the conducting impulse, CardioWave, is capable of solving the system of equations represented by the matrix in parallel. The number of processors that may be used, however, is limited to the matrix size divided by the bandwidth. A matrix with a large bandwidth may thus be run with relatively few processors. The Cuthill-McGee permutation algorithm is used to produce a bandwidth-minimized matrix.

The bandwidth-minimized matrix (A) is used as an input to the CardioWave package.[3,4] CardioWave provides an efficient means of solving the equality Ax = b on parallel computers, where the vector x represents the unknown potentials at a point in time and has a distinct value at each timestep and the vector b incorporates the membrane currents at each point in space and varies with time. CardioWave permits the selection of a variety of modules with which the simulation will be conducted. For instance, the membrane dynamics may be chosen from a number of available models, different solvers and time stepping algorithms may be used, and a variety of output formats are available. Also, a particular stimulus scheme is usually imposed. With these choices made, the simulation may proceed. For large-scale models of atrial activation, simulations were performed on 5 and 40 Power3 200 MHz processors of an IBM SP RS/6000 at the North Carolina Supercomputing Center (Research Triangle Park, NC). The specific number of processors used in each case depended on the matrix bandwidth limitations and the processor availability. The simulation times can be long. For a 243,000-element model simulated for 1.2 seconds and run on 24 processors, 13.5 hours of computation were required.

Output Formats

The selection of the output format in CardioWave determines the form of the results. Three data formats are used most often. In one, the transmembrane potential at a point or several points is dumped, examined directly using a two-dimensional plotting utility. In the second data format, the transmembrane potential at each point in the mesh is outputted as a series of timesteps. Data recorded in this fashion is typically visualized using a custom network in AVS/Express (Advanced Visual Systems, Inc, Waltham, MA). This format has the advantage that it makes available the activity at all points in the mesh at the same time, in an animated sequence. The drawback, however, is the tendency to produce huge datafiles with this output format. The 243,000-element mesh simulated for 1.2 seconds, with output at every msec, generates a 278-megabyte datafile. An MPEG encoded representation of this sequence, on the other hand, consumes only 3.3 megabytes. The last data format is an activation map in which the only the time at which a given point is activated (reaches a predefined potential) is outputted.

Other Considerations

The tissue was represented as a monodomain and the representation is three-dimensional, incorporating both the left and right atria and the major muscle bundles of the atria, including the crista terminalis, pectinate muscles, limbus of the fossa ovalis, and Bachmann's bundle. The bulk tissue is isotropic and the bundles are represented as anisotropic structures with fiber directions aligned with the bundle axes. The ionic fluxes are governed to the human atrial cell formulation of Nygren et al.[5] Table-lookup for some of the rate constants was used to accelerate the calculations. To minimize complexity, only three conductivities are assigned to the model. The values of conductivities were selected to obtain realistic conduction velocities of approximately 60–75 cm/sec in the bulk tissue, 150–200 cm/sec in the bundles and 30–40 cm/sec in slow regions. A first-order, semi-implicit time integration scheme was used with a fixed time step of 20 msec. The system of equations was solved iteratively using the Conjugate Gradient method with a convergence tolerance of 10-6.

Results

The approach outlined above enables the simulation of both normal and abnormal activation using the human atrial model. The normal patterns were validated through qualitative comparison with those reported from experimental mapping studies.[6,7] Figure 2 presents various views of the normal activation sequence on the human atrial model using activation isolines. The color blue represents the early activation and red the late activation. The entire sequence takes about 123 msec. Panel (a) highlights the anisotropic conduction along the crista (A). Note in (b) the circle of activation formed around the first point of breakthrough on the right appendage, at the terminus of the first pectinate muscle (B). This panel also presents a view of the point of last activation of the left atrial appendage (C). In the posterior view (c), the rapid propagation along the intercaval

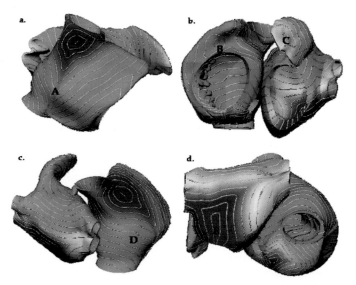

Figure 2. Normal activation sequence from various views of atria. Isolines are 5 msec apart.

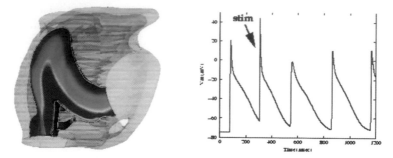

Figure 3. One time step of a cycle of typical atrial flutter showing the transmembrane potential distribution (left). The transmembrane potential as a function time at a site near the second stimulus used to induce the flutter is shown on the right.

bundle causes a slight deflection of the isolines (D). In (d), notice the convergence of the three wavefronts to the point of last atrial activation, in the left atrial posterior inferior tissue (E). The bunched isolines in the right atrial floor reflect the slow conduction velocity there (F).

The model is also capable of simulating flutter-like activity.[2] Such "abnormal" activity is not easily obtained using nominally normal values of conductivity and parameters for the membrane currents. One approach to obtain flutter is to create barriers or boundaries to ensure the flutter pattern is not disrupted. In the model, such boundaries can be created by either making changes to the properties of different sub-blocks or by adding a ridge of insulated or inexcitable tissue (e.g., an incision). One advantage of the model is the ability to monitor spatially the transmembrane potential and ionic changes as the flutter continues (Figure 3).

Conclusions

Using a procedure similar to that used in other disciplines in engineering, we constructed a three-dimensional model of the human atria to study normal and abnormal wavefront conduction. By using multiblock meshing it is possible to add, remove or modify structures to explore their impact on activation. The modular approach also allows for new and/or multiple membrane models or tissue properties to be introduced. Similarly, adding features like the computation of extracellular potentials (for more direct comparison to experiment) is possible, but with additional computational cost. Because of its high level of detail, the present model can be used to determine whether simpler models such as those that represent the atria only as simple surfaces or with reduced membrane models are sufficient to capture important information.

As computers become faster and algorithms more robust, more realistic computers models of the heart can be used to explore how changes at the membrane level interact with changes in tissue properties and geometry to give rise to arrhythmias. However, much work is still needed to determine how best to reduce the enormous amount of data generated from these large-scale models to develop meaningful strategies for therapy. This data reduction process along with new ways to introduce statistical variance in simulation parameters will likely play a critical role in the next generation of biological modeling paradigms.

References

1. Harrild DM, Penland RC, Henriquez CS. A flexible method for simulating cardiac conduction in three-dimensional complex geometries. *J Electrocardiology* 2000;33:241–251.
2. Harrild DM. Why Anatomy Matters: Normal Conduction and Flutter in a Computer Model of the Human Atria. *Ph.D. Thesis*, Duke University, 2000.
3. Pormann JB, Henriquez CS, Board JA, et al. Computer simulations of cardiac electrophysiology, *SuperComputing 2000 Annual Conference.*
4. http://www.ee.duke.edu/~jpormann/simsys/CardioWave.html
5. Nygren A, Fiset C, Firek L, et al. Mathematical model of an adult human atrial cell. The role of K+ currents in repolarization. *Circ Res* 1998;82:63–81.
6. Schuessler RB, Kawamoto T, Hand DW, et al. Simultaneous epicardial and endocardial activation sequence mapping in the isolated canine right atrium. *Circulation* 1993;88:250–263.
7. Harrild DM, Henriquez CS. A computer model of normal conduction in the human atria. *Circ Res* 2000;87:E25–E36.

Chapter 14

Auckland Whole Heart Model:
An Integrated Computational Framework for the Construction of a Whole Organ Model of Cardiac Function

Nicolas P. Smith, PhD, Peter J. Mulquiney, PhD, Denis Noble, PhD, Peter J. Hunter, PhD

Introduction

We present the current state of the model components from our groups necessary to construct a coupled metabolism, electrophysiology and mechanics model of the heart. Within this project, development is on three fronts: 1) the representation of the complex three dimensional structure of ventricular and arterial anatomy 2) the modeling of biophysically-based equations that describe the transient ionic concentration changes at the cellular level and the continuum behaviour for the whole organ 3) the development of software tools at the Universities of Auckland and Oxford that form both the computational framework for each model and also provide an essential way of visualizing complex spatial-temporal data. Finally the model is discussed in relation to the Cardiome, an anatomically based integrated model of cardiac function.

The recent advances in high performance computing together with mathematical modeling now provide a framework for the coupling of previously separate areas of cardiac physiology. Increased computational power means detailed biophysically based models of single cell systems of electrophysiology, contraction and metabolism can begin to be incorporated into two and three dimensional, and ultimately whole organ representations of cardiac tissue. Furthermore, the goal of whole organ research via modeling provides motivation for coupling each of these sys-

From Virag N, Blanc O, Kappenberger L (eds): *Computer Simulation and Experimental Assessment of Cardiac Electrophysiology.* ©Futura Publishing Co., Inc., Armonk, NY, 2001.

tems together, where their complex interactions can be investigated at macroscopic level. The ultimate goal for this work is the ability to accurately predict whole organ behavior under normal and pathological conditions, such as during myocardial ischemia or re-entrant arrhythmias. Outlined in this chapter is the mathematical framework within which the physiological components, being developed in our respective groups, are coupled together. Critical to the interpretation, ongoing development of and communication between these (often large) models are the software environments built specifically to accommodate the non-linearities inherent in biology. Such software has been designed to perform three distinct functions: 1) back-end computations associated with solving finite element approximations in space and time, 2) the three-dimensional visualization of biological data, and 3) the interpretation and exchange of model representations.

Cardiac Anatomy

The anatomically accurate finite element model of the cardiac ventricles forms the basis of the geometric domain over which the continuum equations that govern whole organ behavior are solved. These equations include those of finite deformation which are solved for mechanics stimulations and the advection diffusion equation to simulate propagation. Biophysically based cellular models of electrophysiology[1] and cardiac mechanics[2] are used to calculate the current sources at grid points and active tension at gauss points respectively within each finite element.

The heart model is based on data from careful anatomical studies of canine ventricles by Legrice et al.[3,4] Using nonlinear fitting techniques efficient finite element representations of two geometric fields have been created by Nielsen et al.[5] The first field is the set of geometric variables (prolate spheroidal coordinates λ, μ, θ) which are defined at each node in the finite element mesh. It is this part of the geometric description of the ventricles that defines the myocardial volume. The second field contains the fibrous-sheet orientations throughout the myocardium. This anisotropic structure is an important determinant of ventricular mechanics and activation wave propagation. Each field is fitted in a finite element mesh consisting of 120 high order finite elements and 195 nodes.

Recently the group at the University of Auckland have also undertaken the development of a finite element based model of the atria which is compatible with the existing ventricular model. This model will be used for investigating conduction phenomena originating at the sino-atrial node including atrial fibrillation as well as the valve mechanics associated with ventricular filling.

A model of the coronary network has been generated from measured epicardial vessels and the topological data of Kassab et al.[6] The largest six of eleven generations of arterial vessels were generated discretely using an avoidance algorithm developed to simultaneously minimize global and local cost functions associated with blood supply.[7] Pairs of veins are assumed to be parallel to each arterial vessel. The network geometry was coupled to material points within the anatomically accurate model of the ventricles used for the whole organ activation and mechanics simulations.

A rudimentary model of the Purkinje fiber architecture has also been developed by applying the volume splitting algorithm of Wang et al.[8] to the myocardial volume defined by the ventricular model. Using the Purkinje fiber electrophysiogy cell model of McAllister et al.[9] the sites of initial activation within the myocardium can be predicted.

Cellular Electrophysiology and Tissue Propagation

Mathematical descriptions of inter-cellular and intra-cellular ion transport in cardiac cells have become increasingly complex since the initial work of Noble.[10] The relative sophistication of these models provides an ideal foundation on which to build models of mechanics and metabolism. The most recent cellular models have included representations of many of the subcellular organelles,[1,11–13] such as the diadic space, sarcoplasmic reticulum (SR) and mitochondria, and/or have been focused specifically on individual ion transporters.[14,15] Typical of complete ventricular cell models are the equations developed by Noble et al.[1], consisting of a system of twenty six ordinary differential equations, specifying the rates of change of key cellular ion concentrations, which are themselves dependent on a number of diffusive and energy dependent exchange processes. Much of the cellular modeling work in our groups is based on the electrophysiological model of Noble et al.[1], which describes biophysically based currents that are coupled to the model of cardiac contraction of Hunter et al.[2] via the changes in cytosolic calcium concentration induced by release from the SR.

The transient changes in ion concentrations are solved by integrating the system of equations that define the rate of each cellular reaction through time. This integration is performed using an Adams-Moulton numerical integration method that uses both adaptive step size and order. This scheme is chosen to accommodate the widely varying time scales of the individual currents over the duration of an action potential (e.g., the rapidly varying sodium current up-stroke compared with the relatively slow changing potassium currents). An efficient integration method is less important when solving single cell models where computational expense is small. However, computational efficiency becomes essential when simulating the combined effect of large numbers of cells in multidimensional models of cardiac tissue.

The effect of inhomogeneities on the function of cardiac tissue is clearly beyond the scope of the single cell models. However, by using these cell model equations to provide current sources embedded in a continuum model, many of the spatio-temporal effects of activation wave propagation can be investigated.

Each numerical approximation point in a tissue model is treated as a "black box," whose source/sink characteristics are determined by the complex ion kinetics of the underlying cellular model. The spread of current is then modeled by numerically solving an advection-diffusion equation over this domain of points. Within the tissue model, conductivity and capacitance determine the electrical coupling between approximation points and ultimately the spread of activation throughout the tissue. The anisotropic nature of cardiac tissue means this conductive coupling is represented by a tensor with values that are determined from the tissue micro-structure that has its local axes aligned with the fibre, sheet and sheet-normal directions in the tissue.

The high mesh density required to accurately represent the large changes in spatial ion gradients at the front of a propagating wave in cardiac tissue lends itself to a finite difference solution technique. The relative efficiency of finite difference grid-point calculations compensates for the large number of grid points required. Despite this, the calculation of activation wave spread in the heart is currently not computationally tractable, since it requires an estimated 1.02 TB of disk storage and the solution to 281 billion equations for a single beat. Two potential solutions to this problem are the combining of the finite difference scheme with multigrid methods, and the applying of parallelization techniques.

The use of multi-grid methods[16,17] introduces several levels of increasing grid density, which are recruited based on the need to represent the spatial gradients in each region. A relatively small number of computational points would be used in regions of inactive or refractory tissue. Higher densities, obtained from interpolating currently active points, would be used in regions at, or just ahead of, the wavefront. We estimate this could result in a 95% reduction in the number of active grid points needed at any stage in time, and thus a large computational saving.

The parallelization of grid point calculations is relevant for tissue simulations for two reasons. Firstly, the ionic current calculations at each grid point can be performed independently of those at all other grid points. Second, integrating these complex systems of cellular equations is a major contributor to computational load in comparison to the tissue based differencing scheme. Thus, in theory, large problems should remain linearly scalable for relatively high numbers of processors.

Myocyte and Ventricular Mechanics

Similar to the electrophysiological modeling, active myocardial mechanics have been modeled using a cellular model, which relates transient ionic concentrations to actively developed tension. This cell model is then integrated into a continuum framework and used in combination with the finite element method to predict whole organ deformation throughout the cardiac cycle. This deformation is governed by active and passive mechanical properties of the tissue. The passive mechanical properties are modeled using a constitutive law based on the nonlinear and anisotropic nature of cardiac tissue. The active properties are tightly coupled to cardiac activation and metabolism. It is the electrophysiology of the action potential, or more specifically the associated calcium transient that underlies myocyte contraction on a relatively fast time scale. Generated tension is also dependent on the metabolic processes of energy production within the cell. Thus an ionic model of contraction is essential in the development of a fully integrated cardiac model.

Hunter et al.[2] have recently developed such a model. Like the electrophysiological models, the key rates of ionic (calcium) transport and binding are represented via a system of differential and integral equations. Key elements to this model are the binding and release of Ca^{2+} to troponin-C, tropomyosin kinetics and cross-bridge kinetics. The equation parameters are fitted to steady-state tension-length-Ca^{2+} relations and to transient tension responses to rapid length steps for a variety of experimental preparations. The model is then shown to predict results from a range of other tests including the length response to step changes in load, mechanical frequency response tests. The mechanical state of the cell is clearly affected by the Ca^{2+} transient supplied (primarily) from the sarcoplasmic reticulum release channels but the electromechanical coupling also works the other way as well: mechanical perturbations which alter the release of Ca^{2+} from troponin-C also thereby influence the electrophysiological state of the cell.

Whole ventricle deformation was determined using the finite element method to solve the governing equations of finite deformation elasticity for the ventricular model. Deformations were induced by alterations in intra-cellular calcium concentration and in the left and right ventricular cavity pressures, which were incremented throughout the cardiac cycle starting at a residually stressed unloaded resting state. Each subsequent state was solved as a quasi-static problem using the solution from the previous state as the initial condition. The nonlinear system of finite element equations was solved at each step using Newton's method.

The mechanics model of ventricular contraction is split into four distinct phases, diastole (or inflation), isovolumic contraction, ejection and isovolumic relaxation. Each phase consists of a number of individual me-

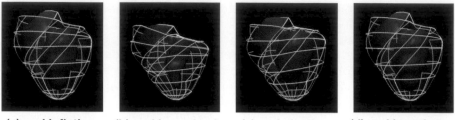

(a) end inflation   (b) end iso-volumic   (c) end ejection   (d) end isovolume
                          contraction   relaxation

Figure 1. The four phases of ventricular mechanics. White lines show the epicardial boundaries of ventricular wall elements, while shaded epicardial surfaces show how the right ventricle wraps around the left ventricle.

chanics steps. The deformation at the end of each phase is shown in Figure 1.

As with the finite difference scheme used to simulate whole organ activation wave propagation, sections of the finite element method algorithm can be divided into blocks on which computations can be performed in parallel. Parallelization of the assembly phase of the global stiffness matrix produced near linear speed up with additional processors, which contributes greatly to reducing overall computation time.

Coronary Blood Flow and Cardiac Energy Production

Coronary blood flow was modeled by assuming a radial axi-symmetric velocity profile, the Navier Stokes equations governing coronary blood flow reduce to one-dimension.[18] These flow equations were combined with a pressure-area relationship for the compliant coronary vessel walls, which has been fitted from experimental data. Blood flow through the coronary network model was calculated using the two-step Lax Wendroff finite difference representation and the coupled lumped parameter model of Smith et al.[18]

The compressive force produced by contraction of the ventricles on the embedded coronary vessels has a major effect on coronary blood flow. This force was calculated from finite element solutions to the finite elasticity equations.[19] For a stress state calculated at a point in the contraction cycle, the stress tensor can be rotated into a vessel coordinate system for each segment in order to calculate the average pressure normal to the vessel wall. This pressure is then incorporated into the pressure-area relationship of the blood flow equations.

Figure 2 demonstrates a central behavior of this modeling study showing calculated arterial coronary blood flow at different stages during the contraction cycle. Despite the rise in arterial inflow pressure during systole, contraction significantly impeded total flow over the whole cycle with flow time integrals less than the steady state values calculated independent of contraction. Along with a number of other key experimental results, this model has been verified using the work of Bassingthwaight et al.[20] on the fractal nature of the regional distribution of blood flow in the heart. What remains is to use this distribution together with metabolic models such that the supply of oxygen determines the nature of energy production and the resulting effects on myocyte and whole heart function.

The main difficulties in modeling metabolism tend to relate to the physiological aspect of the modeling process rather than the mathematics. Mathematically, the task of modeling a metabolic system is relatively simple. As a first approximation, it is usually assumed that metabolite concentrations are spatially homogeneous within each organelle or compartment. Thus, the rates of change of metabolites can be described by a system of ordinary linear differential equations for which the right hand side consists of linear combinations of the rate equations that describe each reaction. Each linear combination is determined by the stoichiometry of the metabolic system. Linear dependencies between the rows of the stoichiometry matrix allow the identification of so called conservation sums, which then allow the elimination of some of the concentration variables from the model. Further simplification can be obtained by a consideration of the time hierarchy of the system. For example, modal analysis can be used to identify the various time scales of the model. This may then allow the use of further approximation methods to again reduce the number of metabolite or state variables.[21]

Cellular metabolism has received extensive experimental study over the last fifty years and much has been learned about the kinetics of the individual metabolic reactions. However, there has been limited success in developing models of metabolism that relate the kinetics of the individual components of the metabolic system to its overall behavior. The only metabolic system for which a detailed and realistic model exists is the human erythrocyte; a cell with a relatively simple metabolism (e.g.,

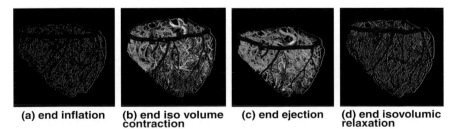

(a) end inflation   (b) end iso volume contraction   (c) end ejection   (d) end isovolumic relaxation

Figure 2. Calculated IMP at the end of the four phases of cardiac mechanics: diastolic loading (or inflation), isovolumic contraction, ejection and isovolumic relaxation.

Mulquiney et al.[22–24]). Part of the reason for this is the immense complexity of metabolic systems; metabolism in the heart consists of a number of highly interrelated pathways that exhibit multi-site regulation by a large number of state variables in a highly nonlinear manner. Only in the last decade or so has the computing power been available to deal with such complicated modeling problems. One early attempt at modeling cardiac metabolism which, to date, remains the most detailed model developed, was the model developed by David Garfinkel and co-workers (e.g., see Garfinkel et al.[25]) and we are currently using this as a basis for a detailed model of cellular metabolism.

In the task of incorporating metabolism into the current cellular models, it has been necessary to modify many of the electrophysiological and mechanics rate equations to account for the interactions of ATP, as well as a number of other metabolites. To do this in a consistent manner, new rate equations have been derived for many processes that are based on a detailed consideration of each reaction mechanism. Many of the existing rate equations were based on equations containing 'apparent' constants, which were only valid for a limited set of conditions. In many pathological conditions, the concentrations of ions and metabolites vary greatly and the use of apparent constants is no longer valid.

Visualization and Computational Software

The Oxsoft software was first released in 1984 as a means of investigating the role of sodium-calcium exchange in calcium efflux, and in arrhythmic mechanisms.[26] PC-based and written in Borland Pascal 7.08, it has since become a critical tool in the development and interpretation of electrophysiology and more recently metabolic models of the single myocyte. The Oxsoft program incorporates a variety of experimental pacing and voltage protocols which enables rapid investigation and analysis of both experimental and modeling results.

CMISS has been developed over the last 20 years in the Department of Engineering Science, University of Auckland, New Zealand, to specifically implement numerical techniques relevant to the mathematical modeling of biological problems. Using **CMISS** multiple high order finite and boundary element solution domains can be coupled together for different problem types solved using a variety of numerical methods. The computational kernel written primarily in Fortran (**CM**) of **CMISS** is used for all major continuum computations. The graphical front end and user interface written in C (**CMGUI**) is used to view and manipulating data within **CMISS**. Within the continuum framework provided by **CMISS** the systems of ordinary differential equations used to represent each cellular model are included and integrated thought time.

An extremely important factor in the development of an integrated software package is the ability to quickly and without errors implement published cellular and continuum models developed to describe each area of cardiac function. To this end the CellML and FieldML standards are being developed.[27] Based on the eXtensible Markup Language (XML), functional units are set up representing individual structures, relationships or useful model groupings. Each unit may consist of local and global variables, data or mathematical relations described using MathML. Connections between units map the global variables from one unit to another and, in doing so, specify the coupling of different aspects of function. There are a multitude of benefits of establishing a common format with which to represent models. Such a representation will be platform-independent and will enforce a consistent set of units (from which fundamental equations can be checked). Based in an internet meta language, models will be able to be transferred quickly between research groups. From the CellML and FieldML representations, text equations for traditional publication or code in a variety of computer languages can be exported which are consistent, thereby eliminating many of the errors to which these complex models are currently prone.

Discussion and Future Developments

The foundation components of a fully integrated and functional model of the heart have been presented. Further work developing and refining elements of the cardiac system remains. On the cellular level, this includes adding further cell types, species models and characterizing responses to pathologies such as ischemia. At the whole organ level, work to refine the anatomical structures of the conduction network is underway, along with adding a model of the ventricular fluid dynamics.

Coupling of these individual models is now much of the focus of work in our respective laboratories. Important to this work is the further development of techniques that span the variety of spatial and, particularly, temporal scales of the many different processes we are attempting to model. For example, the time-scale of the sodium current that initiates an action potential is 1–2 ms. In contrast, the stores of ATP fueling metabolism and contraction take up to 10 minutes to completely deplete from the initial onset of total ischemia.[28] The solution is a hierarchy of models dependent on the processes involved. Fast reactions may need to be reduced to algebraic expressions when modeling the slower metabolic reactions in order to efficiently integrate the system of equations. Conversely, the concentrations of metabolites may be assumed constant for the time-scale, over which individual electrophysiological currents are studied.

Levels of model complexity are also required to fully exploit the wealth of data available from the rapidly expanding fields of molecular-biology and genomics within a currently available computational framework. Using this data, there is real potential to develop cellular models using continuum principles by spatially representing the mechanics of cellular contractile apparatus, ionic diffusion and transport processes. Such models may provide a valuable way to link protein and gene information to cell function. They would, however, in the medium term prove too computationally expensive to be replicated millions of times in a tissue model. Thus, one solution is to provide computationally simple models within the tissue framework, which are based on the more detailed models but still maintain the essential elements of each process.

Critical to any modeling project where different aspects of function are being incorporated together, is constant and systematic experimental verification. As with model development, verification is essential at all levels from protein ion channel characteristics to whole organ function. Such an integrated approach will require input from a wide variety of groups around the world. The development of the Cardiome, as a subset of the Physiome Project initiated by Dr. Jim Bassingthwaighte in 1997, will provide a framework for this cooperative effort. The databases developed through this initiative of experimental data and mathematical models will prove invaluable in expediting this process. It is with this focussed effort that the goal of biophysically based and clinically relevant integrated cardiac modeling will become a reality.

Acknowledgments: We would like to acknowledge the contributions of Dr. David Bullivant, Dr. Poul Nielsen, Dr. Martyn Nash, Dr. Chris Bradley, Dr. Andrew Pullan, Dr. Greg Sands and Martin Buist to the **CMISS** code on which the simulations discussed in this paper are based. The first author is supported by a Post-Doctoral Fellowship from the New Zealand Foundation for Research Science and Technology.

References

1. Noble D, Varghese A, Kohl P, et al. Improved guinea-pig ventricular model incorporating diadic space, i_{kr} and i_{ks} , length and tension-dependent processes. *Can J Cardiol* 1998;14:123–134.
2. Hunter PJ, McCulloch AD, Ter Keurs HEDJ. Modeling the mechanical properties of cardiac muscle. *Prog Biophys Molec Biol* 1998;69:289–331.
3. Le Grice IJ, Smaill BH, Hunter PJ. The laminar myocardium: Implications for ventricular function. *In Biomechanics Conf UCSD*, San Diego (1992).
4. Le Grice IJ, Smaill BH, Hunter PJ. Myocardial activation by threshold modeling with an anatomically accurate finite element model. *In Proc Biomedical Engineering Society* (1992).
5. Nielsen PMF, Le Grice IJ, Smaill BH, et al. Mathematical model of geometry and fibrous structure of the heart. *Am J Physiol* 1991;260:H1365–H1378.

6. Kassab GS, Rider CA, Tang NJ, et al. Topology and dimensions of pig coronary capillary network. *Am J Physiol* 1994;267:H319–H325.

7. Smith NP, Pullan AJ, Hunter PJ. The generation of an anatomically accurate geometric coronary model. *Ann Biomed Eng* 2000;28:14–25.

8. Wang CY, Bassingthwaighte JB, Weissman LJ. Bifurcating distributive system using Monte Carlo method. *Mathl Comput Modeling* 1992;16(3):91–98.

9. McAllister RE, Noble D, Tsien RW. Reconstruction of the electrical activity of cardiac purkinje fibres. *J Physiol* 1975;251:1–59.

10. Noble D. A Modification of the Hodgkin-Huxley equation applicable to Purkinje fibre action and pacemaker potentials. *J Physiol* 1962;160:317–352.

11. Jafri S, Rice J, Winslow R. Cardiac Ca^{2+} dynamics: The role of ryanodine receptor adaptation and sarcoplasmic reticulum load. *Biophys J* 1998;74: 1149–1168.

12. Luo C, Rudy Y. A dynamic model of the cardiac ventricular action potential: I. Simulations of ionic currents and concentration changes. *Circ Res* 1994; 74(6):1071–1096.

13. Luo C, Rudy Y. A dynamic model of the cardiac ventricular action potential: II. Afterdepolarizations, triggered activity, and potentiation. *Circ Res* 1994; 74(6):1097–1113).

14. Rice J, Winslow R, Dekanski J, et al. Model studies of the role of mechano-sensitive currents in the generation of cardiac arrhythmias. *J Theor Biol* 1998; 190:295–312.

15. Snyder S, Palmer B, Moore R. A mathematical model of cardiocyte Ca^{2+} dynamics with a novel representation of sarcoplasmic reticular Ca^{2+} control. *Biophys J* 2000;79:94–115.

16. Briggs WL. **A Multigrid Tutorial**. Society for Industrial and Applied Mathematics, Philadelphia, Pennsylvania, 1987.

17. Sands GB, Hunter PJ. A collocation-multigrid model of bidomain activation as a component of a complete electrocardiology model. *In 23rd International Conference on Electrocardiography* (1996).

18. Smith NP, Pullan AJ, Hunter PJ. An efficient finite difference model of transient coronary blood flow in the heart. *SIAM J Appl Math* 2001 (in press).

19. Nash MP. Mechanics and material properties of the heart using an anatomically accurate mathematical model. *PhD Thesis*, The University of Auckland, New Zealand, 1998.

20. Bassingthwaighte JB, King RB, Roger SA. Fractal nature of regional myocardial blood flow heterogeneity. *Circ Res 1989*;65:578–590.

21. Heinrich R, Schuster S. **The Regulation of Cellular Systems**. Ninth edition. Chapman and Hall, New York, 1996.

22. Mulquiney PJ, Bubb WA, Kuchel PW. Model of 2,3- bisphosphoglycerate metabolism in the human erythrocyte based on detailed enzyme kinetic equations: In-vivo kinetic characterisation of 2,3- bisphosphoglycerate synthase/phosphatase using 13C and 31P NMR. *Biochem J* 1999;342:567–580.

23. Mulquiney PJ, Kuchel PW. Model of 2,3-bisphosphoglycerate metabolism in the human erythrocyte based on detailed enzyme kinetic equations: Computer simulation and metabolic control analysis. *Biochem J* 1999;342:597–604.

24. Mulquiney PJ, Kuchel PW. Model of 2,3-bisphosphoglycerate metabolism in the human erythrocyte based on detailed enzyme kinetic equations: Equations and parameter refinement. *Biochem J* 1999;342:581–596.

25. Garfinkel D, Kohn MC, Achs MJ. Computer simulation of metabolism in pyruvate-purfused rat heart. V. Physiological implications. *Am J Physiol* 1979;237: R181–R186.

26. Noble D, Noble SJ. A model of the sino-atrial node electrical activity based on a modification of the DiFrancesco-Noble (1984) equations. *Proc R Soc London* 1984;222:295–304.

27. Hedley WJ, Nelson MR, Bullivant DP, et al. A short introduction to cellml. *Phil Trans* 2001. (in press).

28. Ch'en FFT, Vaughan-Jones RD, Clark K, et al. Modeling myocardial ischaemia and reperfusion. *Prog Biophys Molec Biol* 1998;69:497–515.

Part V.

Options in the Treatment of Atrial Fibrillation

Chapter 15

Mechanisms of Atrial Fibrillation

Albert L. Waldo, MD

Introduction

For a long time, there has been much speculation, but little detailed understanding of the mechanism of atrial fibrillation (AF). With improvements in technology, particularly in the last two decades, with the development of several animal models, and with new data from patients, we now have come to appreciate that there are probably several mechanisms of AF. And perhaps due to remodeling, the several mechanisms may ultimately evolve to a final common mechanism. The following discussion of mechanisms of AF will be largely chronologic, and will be limited to the mechanisms as we currently understand them. It is likely that a more sophisticated understanding will become appreciated as more research is done.

The Early Studies

In papers published in 1906[1] and 1908,[2] Mayer was the first to elucidate the fundamental principles of reentry. Mayer studied contractions initiated in rings of tissue cut from the bell of the jellyfish (Scyphomedusae). He showed that when he mechanically stimulated the tissue, two contraction waves traveled around the ring in opposite directions from the point of stimulus. When they collided, the contraction waves were extinguished. However, when he applied temporary pressure on only one side of the site of mechanical stimulus, although two contractile waves again

[1] Supported in part by grant # RO1-HL38408 from the National Institutes of Health, National Heart, Lung, and Blood Institute, Bethesda, MD.

From Virag N, Blanc O, Kappenberger L (eds): *Computer Simulation and Experimental Assessment of Cardiac Electrophysiology.* ©Futura Publishing Co., Inc., Armonk, NY, 2001.

were produced, one was blocked at the site of the pressure. The other, however, traveled away from the stimulus in the unblocked direction, and with removal of the pressure (i.e., block), this contraction wave was able to travel continuously around the muscle ring. In fact, it could be maintained for hours or days. From these studies, it was realized that for reentry to occur, the appropriate substrate had to be present, there had to be unidirectional block after initiation of the waves, there needed to be a central area of block (the hole in the ring made from the bell of the jelly fish) around which the reentry wave could circulate, and conduction time around the circuit had to exceed the refractory period. It was Mines who recognized the potential application of these observations to clinical arrhythmias. In 1913, he extended Mayer's work to the atria of turtles, frogs, and electric rays. He showed that in these atria, just as in Mayer's Scyphomedusae, a circus movement of contractile waves could be induced.[3] He showed that the refractory period was inversely related to stimulation rate, and characterized the impact of wavelength (conduction velocity x refractory period) on fibrillation.

However, for the specific study of AF, a major challenge was the difficulty in creating suitable animal models. As recognized by Lewis et al.,[4] there was an inability to produce sustained tachyarrhythmias in normal canine atria, and a technical inability to map AF even if it lasted for any period. As we now know, to make sustained AF in the canine heart and other mammalian hearts of moderate size, abnormal (pathological) conditions resulting from interventions such as application of substances, vagal stimulation, prolonged rapid pacing, heart failure, or inflammation usually must first be imposed.

Nevertheless, based on observations of dying hearts made without any electrophysiological or even mechanical recordings, Garrey, in a seminal paper published in 1914,[5] established the fundamental concept that a critical mass of tissue was necessary to maintain fibrillation of any sort (atrial or ventricular). He induced AF by introducing Faradic stimulation at the tip of one of the atrial appendages. When he separated the tip of the appendage from the fibrillating atria, he found that "as a result of this procedure, the appendage came to rest, but the auricles invariably continued their delirium unaltered." From such observations, Garrey concluded that "any small auricular piece will cease fibrillating even though the excised pieces retained their normal properties." Also, based on his studies, and influenced by the work of Mayer and Mines, Garrey later proposed[6] that AF was due to". . . a series of ring-like circuits of shifting location and multiple complexity." Interestingly enough, this is now one of the demonstrated mechanisms of AF.[7] Subsequently, Lewis,[8,9] also influenced by Mayer and Mines, proposed a similar mechanism, namely that, "In fibrillation . . . a single circus movement does exist, but the path changes . . . grossly; but in general the same broad path is used over and over again. *A priori* it is possible to conceive of circus movements of many types. We might even assume several circuits, completely or transiently independent of each other, and each controlling for a time material sections of the muscle . . ." However, Lewis felt "that [in AF] the most mass of muscle is animated by a single circus movement . . . varying with limits . . ." As we shall see, such a mechanism of AF also now has been demonstrated.[10,11]

In the mid 1940s, on the basis of estimates of the velocity of potential circulating reentrant wave fronts of excitation, Wiener and Rosenbleuth[12] calculated that some anatomical orifices (entry and exit points of the great vessels and pulmonary veins) were too small to permit sustained reentrant excitation. However, they suggested that the orifice of the inferior vena cava might be large enough to sustain reentrant atrial flutter, and they inferred that the smaller orifice of the superior vena cava would serve for AF. They also mentioned "the possibility that the pulmonary veins, singly or jointly, may provide effective obstacles for flutter or fibrillation." Two important assumptions were implicit in this work. Assumption #1, similar to the hypotheses of Garrey[6] and Lewis,[8] was that AF could be due to a single reentrant circuit generating a rhythm of such short cycle length that the remainder of the atria cannot follow 1:1. The latter we now call fibrillatory conduction, and the first assumption *in toto* appears to be one of the AF mechanisms. Assumption #2, also implicit in the early studies, including those of Lewis,[4] was that conduction velocity in the reentrant circuit was constant. This second assumption is usually not operative, as functional or anatomical areas of slow conduction are the rule in almost all reentrant circuits.

As can be seen from the above, explicit or implicit in most of the early studies was the notion that if a reentrant circuit was responsible for an arrhythmia, the reentry wavefront traveled around an anatomical obstacle, such as a vessel orifice. However, in the 1970s, Allessie and colleagues[13–15] demonstrated in the isolated left atrium of rabbit hearts that reentrant excitation could occur in which the center of the reentrant circuit was functionally determined. This form of reentry was called "leading circle reentry."[15] It was an important advance in our understanding of reentry and our subsequent appreciation that functionally determined reentrant circuits of very short cycle length might generate AF.

Development of Controversy: Is Atrial Fibrillation Due to Reentry or a Single Focus Firing Rapidly?

Support for the concept that AF may result from a single focus firing rapidly initially came from the work from Scherf and colleagues,[16–18] later repeated by others.[19,20] They placed aconitine on the atria and demonstrated that both a rapid, regular, atrial rhythm consistent with atrial flutter; and a rapid, irregular, atrial rhythm consistent with AF could be generated from a single focus firing rapidly. When the site of aconitine application was excluded by cooling, clamping or removal, the tachycardia terminated. Additionally, it was suggested that the degree of rapidity of firing at the aconitine site determined whether the rhythm generated was atrial flutter or AF. Subsequent studies by Goto et al.[21] and Azuma et al.[22] found that aconitine placed on rabbit atria indeed causes a very rapid rate, apparently due to abnormal automaticity. These findings demonstrate that a single focus firing rapidly (whatever the cause) is capable of producing AF. It is assumed that the impulses generated from the aconitine site occur so rapidly that the atria cannot follow in a 1:1 fashion. The result is fibrillatory conduction causing AF. This old concept was originally not widely accepted. However, it now appears that a single focus firing rapidly regardless of the cause (e.g., reentry, automaticity, or rapid pacing) not only is capable of generating AF, but also is the dominant mechanism of AF, present in most contemporary animal models, and now even in patients.[23–26]

Since the studies of Nahum and Hoff,[27] it has been known that cholinergic stimulation can produce AF in the canine heart, either alone or in association with premature beats. In 1959, largely based on studies of a vagally mediated model of AF and the aconitine induced model of AF, both in the canine heart, Moe and Abildskov proposed the multiple wavelet hypothesis, in which random reentry was the cause of AF.[20,21] AF was postulated to consist of a critical number of randomly distributed reentrant wavelets. The pathways of these wavelets were not anatomically determined, but rather were determined by the local atrial refractoriness and excitability. Because of this, the wavelets could collide and annihilate, divide, or fluctuate in size and velocity. Importantly, little or no head-tail interaction (i.e., circus movement) was present during this type of reentry.

Moe and Abildskov considered the multiple reentrant wavelet hypothesis to be one of several competing mechanisms which could explain the observed properties of AF. Alternative mechanisms which they suggested could underlie high rate atrial activation included: 1) a single ectopic focus firing rapidly, 2) multiple ectopic foci firing rapidly, and 3) a single reentrant impulse around a fixed circuit. Moe favored the multiple reentrant wavelet hypothesis because it could best explain the stability of episodes of AF, which he recognized could last for years in some individuals.[28] In one of the earliest computer simulations of an arrhythmia, Moe and colleagues were able to demonstrate that the multiple reentrant wavelet model could reproduce many of the features of AF in animals or man.[29] However, his model predicted that a large number (>30) of circulating reentrant wavelets were necessary to sustain AF. The subsequent experimental work in the canine atria of Allessie, et al.[30] has shown that far fewer wavelets (4 to 6) were required to sustain AF (c.f.).

Multisite Mapping and Experimental Models of Sustained Atrial Fibrillation

The next advances in our understanding of AF resulted from the combination of the use of simultaneous multi-site mapping techniques to analyze activation of the atria, and the development of new models in which AF was sustained. Allessie and colleagues[30,31] developed a Langendorff-perfused canine atrial model of AF. In this model, sustained AF was produced by rapid atrial pacing during infusion of acetylcholine. When the pacing was stopped, AF persisted as long as the acetylcholine was infused. During the study, endocardial atrial electrograms were recorded simultaneously from a selection of 192 of the 960 electrodes present in specially designed electrode "eggs" inserted through the tricuspid and mitral valve orifices. Analysis of the activation maps during AF demonstrated multiple, simultaneously circulating reentrant wavelets of the random reentry type, although they also occasionally described reentry with head-tail interaction (i.e., circus movement). These studies provided the proof that the multiple reentrant wavelet hypothesis proposed by Moe and Abildskov could be a cause of AF.[20]

More recently, several other models have been described. An *in vitro* canine right atrial model described by Schuessler et al.[32] was shown to have a functionally determined figure-of-eight reentrant circuit of very short cycle length (45 ms) induced by rapid pacing during acetylcholine infusion. The very short cycle length of the reentrant circuit generated fibrillatory conduction, i.e., an AF rhythm, in the remainder of the preparation. Thus, once again, the concept of a single focus producing a rapid rhythm which the atria cannot follow 1:1 (fibrillatory conduction) was operative.

A third model of AF was developed by Cox and colleagues[33] by creating mitral regurgitation in the canine heart. This model is difficult to produce, and is associated with a high mortality rate. Simultaneous multi-site mapping studies ". . . exhibited a spectrum of abnormal patterns ranging from the simplest pattern, in which a single reentrant circuit was present that activated the remainder of the atria, to the most complex cases, in which no consistent pattern of activation could be identified." Although septal activation maps were not obtained, and mapping for longer periods during AF are needed to characterize this model further, the presence of unstable reentrant circuits of short cycle length during AF suggest, once again, that fibrillatory conduction is an important mechanism of AF.

A fourth model of AF is the canine sterile pericarditis model,[7,34] suggested by observation of patients with atrial flutter and AF in the immediate post-operative period following open-heart surgery. AF is induced by rapid atrial pacing or programmed atrial pacing 1 to 2 days after surgically creating the pericarditis. On postoperative days 3 and 4, the inducibility of AF decreases, principally because atrial flutter is induced.[7,34] Simultaneous multisite mapping studies have shown that, in this model, AF is produced by either of 2 mechanisms. One is due to multiple unstable reentrant circuits of very short cycle length which drive the atria at rates which cannot be followed in a 1:1 fashion (fibrillatory conduction). In the latter example, the reentrant circuits are short lived (mean 3–4 rotations), but subsequently are reformed so that 1–4 (mean 1.4 per 100 ms window) unstable reentrant circuits are always present.[7] The other mechanism is a single, stable reentrant circuit of very short cycle length, generally traveling around one or more pulmonary veins, which generates fibrillatory conduction to the remainder of the atria.[10]

A fifth model of AF, also in the canine heart, is the continuous vagal stimulation model used by Moe and Abildskov,[20] in which AF is initially induced by a burst of rapid atrial pacing.[35–37] Although not fully characterized, the mechanism of maintenance of AF in this model has been suggested to be due to unstable reentrant circuits.[35]

A sixth model of AF is that produced simply by various forms of rapid pacing. Sustained or intermittent rapid atrial pacing in canine and goat hearts, respectively[38,39] has been shown to induce AF. While these models are still being characterized, demonstration of consistent pathophysiological changes (shortening of the atrial effective refractory period, and histological changes consistent with hibernation) resulting from the persistent rapid atrial rate has already led to the appreciation that "atrial fibrillation begets atrial fibrillation." This important concept has enormous implications for understanding the progressive nature of AF,[39] as does the fact that these changes appear to be reversible, at least after 2–4 weeks of AF. In sheep, pacing the atria rapidly for a brief period results in AF that persists for relatively long periods.[11,40,41] This model also remains to be characterized more fully, but already has been shown to produce either a single rotor (reentrant circuit) in the left atrium which causes fibrillatory conduction in the right atrium[11] or spiral wave reentry in the right atrium.

As AF is a frequent complication of heart failure, several pacing induced heart failure models of AF have been developed. Following high rate (190 bpm) continuous pacing of the ventricles of sheep, a pacing induced cardiomyopathy diminishes ventricular performance.[42] In this condition, there is a significant increase in the susceptibility of the atria to the induction of AF. Two other models of AF in conjunction with pacing induced heart failure have been recently described. One is a canine model in which the ventricles are paced rapidly for several weeks, after which atrial pacing can induce an atrial tachycardia due to a single focus firing rapidly. This focus is usually in the region of the pulmonary veins, but can also be found in the right atrium, and seems to be due to delayed afterdepolarizations.[43] When the atria can no longer follow the high rate of the atrial tachycardia, or if an atrial extrastimulus is given, atrial fibrillation is initiated. Another model is one created by infusing microspheres into the coronary arteries.[44] This causes global ventricular dysfunction and stable AF once it has been initiated either spontaneously or with pacing. The mechanism of the latter is not yet characterized.

The atrial electrophysiological changes associated with *ventricular* pacing and heart failure in the canine model may be distinct from those caused by AF induced with rapid *atrial* pacing. In further characterization of this model, it has been reported that the atrial effective refractory period (ERP) is actually increased (as opposed to a reduction in response to rapid atrial pacing) prior to the initiation of AF.[45] In addition, the extent of atrial fibrosis was also dramatically increased (0.3% in control, up to ~15% in the animals in congestive heart failure), presumably leading to conduction defects. There was no change in the heterogeneity of refractoriness or conduction velocity at a cycle length of 360 ms.[45]

Studies of Atrial Fibrillation in Patients

Of interest, although rapid atrial pacing animal models of AF are now well established, a study by Moreira et al.[46] in a patient before the era of catheter ablation was the first to show that continuous, long duration rapid atrial pacing could produce persistent atrial fibrillation. In a patient who presented with sustained atrial tachycardia with a resultant tachycardia mediated cardiomyopathy and class IV heart failure, Moreira et al. first showed that burst rapid atrial pacing could produce atrial fibrillation with an easy to control ventricular response rate. However, in the absence of continuous rapid atrial pacing, the atrial tachycardia with 1:1 AV conduction soon returned. Moreira et al. then implanted a permanent rapid atrial pacemaker which paced the atria continuously, initiating and maintaining AF. Control of the ventricular rate was again easily obtained and maintained. The patient's heart function improved to class II, and when the pacing was stopped after a prolonged period (months), the AF had become permanent.

There are several studies in patients which, though limited, were performed in the mapping era, and have been informative. Cox et al.[33] induced AF in patients who had undergone surgical ablation of an accessory AV connection (Wolff-Parkinson-White syndrome) and showed in limited mapping studies that a single unstable reentrant circuit was present in some instances, and an uncertain mechanism, possibly multiple reentrant wavelets, was present in other instances. Konings et al.[47] mapped part of the right and left atrial free walls during AF, also induced in patients after surgical ablation of an accessory AV connection. In the latter studies, three patterns of activation in the right atrial free wall were seen. One included an unstable reentrant circuit. The other two did not really permit a mechanism to be discerned, although one was consistent with multiple-reentrant circuits.

Most recently, using endocardial catheter electrode mapping techniques, Haissaguerre and colleagues have shown in a cohort of patients with paroxysmal AF but without structural heart disease that AF was often generated by a single focus, principally in one of the pulmonary veins, which fired rapidly and generated AF.[26] This has now been widely confirmed, but the mechanism of the impulses generated at these foci is not yet characterized. Furthermore, it is not clear if these foci simply initiate AF in a "favorable atrial substrate" or if these foci continuously drive the atria, generating fibrillatory conduction and clinical AF. Ablation of the responsible focus results in disappearance of the AF. However, the presently reported recurrence rate following ablative treatment of this AF is quite high, as high as 60%. Clearly, there is still much to learn about this intriguing and important mechanism of AF. And adding to the intrigue, as yet there is no experimental counterpart.

Finally in patients, there is the mechanism of tachycardia-induced tachycardia. It has been recognized for many years that atrioventricular reentrant tachycardias (AVRT), atrioventricular nodal reentrant tachycardias (AVNRT), and atrial flutter may be associated with the initiation of AF, and that suppression or cure of the AVRT, AVNRT or atrial flutter is associated with the disappearance of the AF. However, the mechanism of this association is unclear. One possibility is that these arrhythmias facilitate AF by changing the atrial substrate in ways that make the atria more susceptible to AF.[48] An example of facilitation might be that the shortening of the atrial refractory period and other remodeling changes secondary to the rapid atrial rate associated with the initial tachycardia may permit exit of a pulmonary vein focus and thereby trigger AF in an atrial substrate made receptive to it by the preceding tachycardia.

Summary

We are still early in our understanding of AF and its mechanisms. On the basis of what we already have learned from studies of AF in animal models and in patients, there are several mechanisms of AF. Surprisingly, perhaps, the most common mechanism seems to be that of a very rapid focus of some sort (reentrant, autonomic, or triggered) that drives the atria, producing fibrillatory conduction. AF due to multiple reentrant wavelets has only been shown in one model. The best documented mechanism of AF in patients is that due to a pulmonary vein focus firing rapidly. What happens to any initial AF mechanism during AF of very long duration (months-to-years) is not known. With techniques of simultaneous multi-site mapping and other new technologies, new studies should continue to provide the requisite insights and understanding of AF to improve our understanding of AF mechanisms, and, thereby, advance patient care.

References

1. Mayer AG. **Rhythmical Pulsation in Scyphomedusae**. Washington, D.C., Carnegie Institution of Washington. 1906;47:1–62.
2. Mayer AG. **Rhythmical Pulsation in Scyphomedusae. II**. Papers from the Tortugas Laboratory of the Carnegie Institution of Washington 1908;I:113–131.
3. Mines GR. On dynamic equilibrium in the heart. *J Physiol (London)* 1913; 46:349–383.
4. Lewis T, Feil HS, Stroud WD. Observations upon flutter and fibrillation. II, The nature of auricular flutter. *Heart* 1920;7:191–245.
5. Garrey W. The nature of fibrillatory contraction of the heart: Its relation to tissue mass and form. *Am J Physiol* 1914;33:397–414.
6. Garrey WE. Auricular fibrillation. *Physiol Rev* 1924;4:215–250.
7. Kumagai K, Khrestian C, Waldo AL. Simultaneous multisite mapping studies during induced atrial fibrillation in the sterile pericarditis model. Insights into the mechanism of its maintenance. *Circulation* 1997;95:511–521.
8. Lewis T. **The Mechanism and Graphical Registration of the Heart Beat. 3rd ed**, London, Shaw and Sons, Ltd., 1925.
9. Lewis T. Observations upon flutter and fibrillation. IV: Impure flutter; theory of circus movement. *Heart* 1920;7:293–345.
10. Matsuo K, Tomita Y, Uno K, et al. A new mechanism of sustained atrial fibrillation: Studies in the canine sterile pericarditis model. *Circulation* 1998; 98(I):209.
11. Skanes AC, Mandapati R, Berenfeld O, et al. Spatiotemporal periodicity during atrial fibrillation in the isolated sheep heart. *Circulation* 1998;98: 1236–1248.
12. Weiner N, Rosenblueth A. The mathematical formulation of the problem of conduction of impulses in a network of connected excitable elements, specifically in cardiac muscle. *Arch Inst Cardiol Mex* 1946;16:205–265.
13. Allessie MA, Bonke FI, Schopman FJ. Circus movement in rabbit atrial muscle as a mechanism of trachycardia. *Circ Res* 1973;33:54–62.
14. Allessie MA, Bonke FI, Schopman FJ. Circus movement in rabbit atrial muscle as a mechanism of tachycardia. II. The role of nonuniform recovery of excitability in the occurrence of unidirectional block, as studied with multiple microelectrodes. *Circ Res* 1976;39:168–177.
15. Allessie MA, Bonke FI, Schopman FJ. Circus movement in rabbit atrial muscle as a mechanism of tachycardia. III. The "leading circle" concept: A new model of circus movement in cardiac tissue without the involvement of an anatomical obstacle. *Circ Res* 1977;41:9–18.
16. Scherf D. Studies on auricular tachycardia caused by aconitine administration. *Proc Exp Biol Med* 1947;64:233–239.

17. Scherf D, Romano FJ, Terranova R. Experimental studies on auricular flutter and auricular fibrillation. *Am Heart J* 1958;36:241–251.
18. Scherf D, Terranova R. Mechanism of auricular flutter and fibrillation. *Am J Physiol* 1949;159:137–142.
19. Kimura E, Kato K, Murao S, et al. Experimental studies on the mechanism of auricular flutter. *Tohoku J Exp Med* 1954;60:197–207.
20. Moe GK, Abildskov JA. Atrial fibrillation as a self-sustained arrhythmia independent of focal discharge. *Am Heart J* 1959;58:59–70.
21. Goto M, Sakamoto Y, Imanaga I. Aconitine-induced fibrillation of the different muscle tissues of the heart and the action of acetylcholine, in Sano T, Matsuda K, Mizuhira B (eds): **Electrophysiology and Ultrastructure of the Heart**. New York, Grune & Stratton, 1967, pp 199–209.
22. Azuma K, Iwane H, Ibukiyama C, et al. Experimental studies on aconitine-induced atrial fibrillation with microelectrodes. *Isr J Med Sci* 1969;5:470–474.
23. Waldo AL, MacLean WA, Karp RB, et al. Continuous rapid atrial pacing to control recurrent or sustained supraventricular tachycardias following open heart surgery. *Circulation* 1976;54:245–250.
24. Moreira DA, Shepard RB, Waldo AL. Chronic rapid atrial pacing to maintain atrial fibrillation: Use to permit control of ventricular rate in order to treat tachycardia induced cardiomyopathy. *Pac Clin Electrophysiol* 1989;12: 761–775.
25. Waldo AI, Cooper TB. Spontaneous onset of type I atrial flutter in patients. *J Am Coll Cardiol* 1996;28:707–712.
26. Haissaguerre M, Jais P, Shah DC, et al. Spontaneous initiation of atrial fibrillation by ectopic beats originating in the pulmonary veins. *N Engl J Med* 1998;339:659–666.
27. Hoff HE, Geddes LA. Cholinergic factor in auricular fibrillation. *J Appl Physiol* 1955;8:177–192.
28. Moe GK. A conceptual model of atrial fibrillation. *J Electrocardiol* 1968;1: 145–146.
29. Moe GK, Rheinbolt WC, Abildskov JA. A computer model of atrial fibrillation. *Am Heart J* 1964;67:200–220.
30. Allessie MA, Lammers WJEP, Bonke FIM, et al. Experimental evaluation of Moe's multiple wavelet hypothesis of atrial fibrillation, in Zipes DP, Jalife J (eds): **Cardiac Electrophysiology and Arrhythmias**. Orlando, FL, Grune & Stratton, 1985, pp 265–276.
31. Allessie MA, Lammers W, Smeets J, Bonke F, et al. Total mapping of atrial excitation during acetylcholine-induced atrial flutter and fibrillation in the isolated canine heart, in Kulbertus HE, Olsson SB, Schlepper M (eds): **Atrial Fibrillation**. Molndal, Sweden, A.B. Hassle, 1982, pp 44–59.
32. Schuessler RB, Grayson TM, Bromberg BI, et al. Cholinergically mediated tachyarrhythmias induced by a single extrastimulus in the isolated canine right atrium. *Circ Res* 1992;71:1254–1267.
33. Cox JL, Canavan TE, Schuessler RB, et al. The surgical treatment of atrial fibrillation. II. Intraoperative electrophysiologic mapping and description of the electrophysiologic basis of atrial flutter and atrial fibrillation. *J Thorac Cardiovasc Surg* 1991;101:406–426.

34. Pagé PL, Plumb VJ, Okumura K, et al. A new animal model of atrial flutter. *J Am Coll Cardiol* 1986;8:872–879.
35. Wang Z, Pagé P, Nattel S. Mechanism of flecainide's antiarrhythmic action in experimental atrial fibrillation. *Circ Res* 1992;71:271–287.
36. Wang J, Bourne GW, Wang Z, et al. Comparative mechanisms of antiarrhythmic drug action in experimental atrial fibrillation. Importance of use-dependent effects on refractoriness. *Circulation* 1993;88:1030–1044.
37. Wang J, Liu L, Feng J, et al. Regional and functional factors determining induction and maintenance of atrial fibrillation in dogs. *Am J Physiol* 1996;271:H148–H158.
38. Morillo CA, Klein GJ, Jones DL, et al. Chronic rapid atrial pacing. Structural, functional, and electrophysiological characteristics of a new model of sustained atrial fibrillation. *Circulation* 1995;91:1588–1595.
39. Wijffels MC, Kirchhof CJ, Dorland R, et al. Atrial fibrillation begets atrial fibrillation. A study in awake chronically instrumented goats. *Circulation* 1995;92:1954–1968.
40. Powell AC, Garan H, McGovern BA, et al. Low energy conversion of atrial fibrillation in the sheep. *J Am Coll Cardiol* 1992;20:707–711.
41. Ayers GM, Alferness CA, Ilina M, et al. Ventricular proarrhythmic effects of ventricular cycle length and shock strength in a sheep model of transvenous atrial defibrillation. *Circulation* 1994;89:413–422.
42. Power JM, Beacom GA, Alferness CA, et al. Susceptibility to atrial fibrillation: A study in an ovine model of pacing-induced early heart failure. *J Cardiovasc Electrophysiol* 1998;9:423–435.
43. Stambler BS, Shepard RK, Turner DA, et al. Evidence of triggered activity as the mechanism of atrial tachycardia in dogs with pacing-induced heart failure. *J Am Coll Cardiol* 1997;29:254A. Abstract.
44. Nabih MA, Prcevski P, Fromm BS, et al. Effect of ibutilide, a new class III agent, on sustained atrial fibrillation in a canine model of acute ischemia and myocardial dysfunction induced by microembolization. *Pac Clin Electrophysiol* 1993;16:1975–1983.
45. Li D, Fareh S, Leung TK, et al. Promotion of atrial fibrillation by heart failure in dogs: Atrial remodeling of a different sort. *Circulation* 1999;100:87–95.
46. Moreira DA, Shepard RB, Waldo AL. Chronic rapid atrial pacing to maintain atrial fibrillation: Use to permit control of ventricular rate in order to treat tachycardia induced cardiomyopathy. *Pacing Clin Electrophysiol* 1989;12:761–775.
47. Konings KT, Smeets JL, Penn OC, et al. Configuration of unipolar atrial electrograms during electrically induced atrial fibrillation in humans. *Circulation* 1997;95:1231–1241.
48. Allessie MA, Boyden PA, Camm AJ, et al. Pathophysiology and prevention of atrial fibrillation. *Circulation* 2001;103:769–777.

Chapter 16

A Computer Model to Test Therapeutic Interventions for Atrial Fibrillation

Nathalie Virag, PhD, Olivier Blanc, MS,
Olaf Eick, PhD, Jean-Marc Vesin, PhD,
Lukas Kappenberger, MD

Introduction

If they are based on physiological and anatomical parameters, computer models can help us to better understand pathophysiological processes, which are difficult to study in nature, and thereby improve their treatment. Based on ionic current kinetics and taking into account simplified anatomic properties, we developed a computer model of human atria having a three-dimensional structure of one layer of cells. This model realistically simulated atrial arrhythmias during several seconds of real time, with reasonable computation time on standard PCs.

After initiating sustained atrial arrhythmias in the computer model, it is possible to perform an evaluation of different therapeutic interventions. Pacing can be simulated by injecting intracellular current in selected areas. Using this technique it is possible to simulate and study the effect of antitachycardia pacing, preventive pacing, and biatrial or multisite pacing. Defibrillation shocks can be simulated for various electrode configurations, different waveforms and timing. Pharmacological interventions can be tested by an appropriate modulation of the ionic channels. Abla-

[1] This study was made possible by grants from the Theo-Rossi-Di-Montelera Foundation, Medtronic Europe and the Swiss Governmental Commission of Innovative Technologies (CTI).

From Virag N, Blanc O, Kappenberger L (eds): *Computer Simulation and Experimental Assessment of Cardiac Electrophysiology.* ©Futura Publishing Co., Inc., Armonk, NY, 2001.

tion lines, either perfect conduction blocks or incomplete lines, can be easily introduced. Finally, hybrid techniques can also be tested. In this chapter we will focus on ablation since it is the easiest therapy to simulate in our computer model.

In order to obtain data comparable to clinical experiments performed on several patients, and due to the statistical nature of atrial arrhythmias, it is necessary to evaluate each therapeutic strategy in different situations during several seconds of real time, implying several hours or even days of computer time. Time constraint therefore limits the complexity of the computer model. We show here what this implies for the study of ablation lines for atrial fibrillation (AF).

Radiofrequency Ablation

Since atrial flutter is normally due to a single reentrant wave, radiofrequency (RF) ablation can achieve a primary success rate of 85% in humans.[1] On the other hand, AF consists of multiple reentrant waves, so the mechanism of ablation is less clearly understood.[2] One reason is the fact that scientific results obtained in animal models sometimes differ from the clinical experiments. We could therefore use our model of human atria to understand and optimize the complex surgical or RF ablation procedures used for AF. The simulation of linear atrial lesions with a computer model has already been proposed in simpler models.[3]

The surgical Maze procedure has been proved effective in curing AF.[4] More recently, catheter-based RF ablation has been introduced to reproduce the surgical procedure in a less invasive way and different lesion concepts have been suggested.[5,6] However, the optimal composition of lesion lines remains unknown. In the present study, we use our computer model of AF to evaluate the efficacy of different lesion patterns to terminate AF.

The computer model of human atria has been described in great detail in Chapter 3. Perfect ablation lines can be simulated in any location by modifying the conduction (via the resistivity) of the cardiac cells located on the ablation line.

Simulation Results

We tested the effectiveness on AF of seven lesion patterns presented in Figure 1. AF was first induced by the application of two critically timed and located extrastimuli and AF did not terminate spontaneously during the maximum simulation time of 15 seconds. Then, the seven lesion pat-

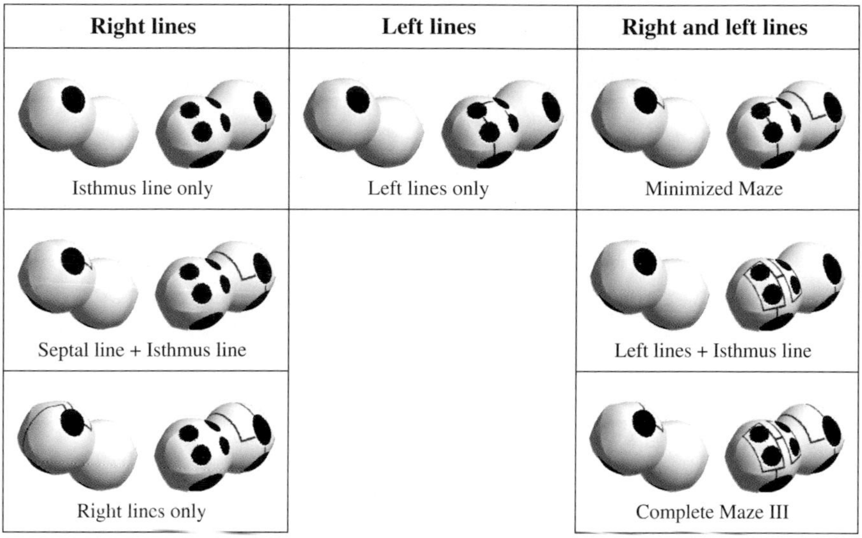

Right lines	Left lines	Right and left lines
Isthmus line only	Left lines only	Minimized Maze
Septal line + Isthmus line		Left lines + Isthmus line
Right lines only		Complete Maze III

Figure 1. Representation of the seven RF lesion patterns that were tested on AF. Veins and valves are represented in black. In each case, on the left is an anterior view with the right atrium on the left, and on the right is the posterior view with the right atrium on the right.

terns were applied at different moments (from 1 to 10 seconds after the start of AF). Therefore, for each lesion pattern, 10 different simulations were performed and the results were averaged. For each simulation, we measured the time until conversion of AF to sinus rhythm or to uncommon atrial flutter. If AF was still running after 6 seconds, we assumed that the ablation pattern was ineffective. Results obtained from the 70 simulations are summarized in Table 1.

In clinical experiments, the Maze procedure cured AF in 89% of patients without the need of antiarrhythmic medication, and is the

Table 1
Computer Simulation of Ablation of AF: Percentage of Sinus Rhythm, Atrial Flutter and AF, and Average Time to Termination or Conversion

Ablation Pattern	Sinus Rhythm (Time to Termination)	AF	Uncommon Atrial Flutter (Time to Flutter)
Complete Maze III	70% (1.5 s ± 0.2 s)	0%	30% (1.2 s ± 0.5 s)
Right lines only	80% (2.3 s ± 1.2 s)	0%	20% (1.9 s ± 0.8 s)
Septal line + Isthmus line	70% (2.3 s ± 0.9 s)	10%	20% (1.9 s ± 0.7 s)
Minimized Maze	40% (3.1 s ± 1.3 s)	0%	60% (2.7 s ± 1.7 s)
Left lines +Isthmus line	60% (2.0 s ± 0.8 s)	20%	20% (3.0 s ± 0.4 s)
Left lines only	30% (2.2 s ± 0.4 s)	50%	20% (1.7 s ± 0.2 s)
Isthmus line only	20% (3.4 s ± 0.2 s)	50%	30% (2.6 s ± 0.7 s)

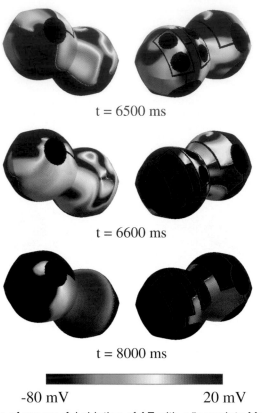

t = 6500 ms

t = 6600 ms

t = 8000 ms

-80 mV   20 mV

Figure 2. Example of successful ablation of AF with a "complete Maze III" lesion pattern. The ablation lesions are applied after 6.5 seconds of AF (first image) and AF is converted into sinus rhythm after 2 seconds.

most effective pattern.[6] In our simulations the complete Maze, right atrial lines and minimized Maze terminated AF. Figure 2 shows an example of how AF is terminated by the application of the complete Maze III lesion pattern. This example shows how the multiple wavelets present during AF are gradually combined into a macroreentrant wave, which then dies because its pathway is blocked. However, it seems that some lesion patterns, even though they terminate AF, are more likely to sustain uncommon atrial flutter (the minimized Maze for example).

In this study, we ran 70 simulations for an average of 8 seconds real time each, more than 9 minutes real time in total. In this case we used a model comprising 65,000 nodes (spatial discretization of 400 μm) with a computation time of 4 hours per second of real time on a Pentium III PC. Total computation time for this study is approximately 93 days with one

PC, or 9–10 days with 10 PCs. Even with such a long simulation time, we observe a great variability in the results, which suggests that we should perform more simulations.

Discussion and Limitations

As in the clinical results, computer simulations show that the Maze procedure is the most efficient in curing AF. It interrupts most of the potential pathways for macroreentrant circuits and consists of multiple atrial incisions. The major problem with this technique is the long procedure time. Our computer model could help find the optimal configuration of right and left lesion lines to replace the Maze procedure with a smaller number of lines, thereby leading to a reduced damage to the atria and reducing the operation time.

The main limitations of this study are firstly that our model takes into account only atrial orifices but not inhomogeneities in the atrial tissue. Secondly, we simulated here only arrhythmias presenting as reentrant multiple wavelets, and did not take into account focal forms of AF (ectopic beats originating mainly from the pulmonary veins in the left atrium[7]). Furthermore, in our computer model the maintenance of AF needs a critical mass, which is provided by the right atrium. This property could explain the good success rate of right-sided lines in ablating AF. As mentioned earlier, computation time is also a strong limitation.

Another problem related to the RF ablation technique is that it is difficult to create ablation lines achieving a complete conduction block and especially to validate the created lines. The computer model could therefore also evaluate the impact of incomplete lines during RF ablation for AF. Finally, it would be interesting to evaluate RF ablation lines together with other therapeutic techniques such as drugs or defibrillation.[3]

This study shows that due to the high number of simulations that must be performed to test different therapies, computer models with simplified features such as the one presented here are needed, allowing a tractable computation time. More detailed models of anatomy and electrophysiology are still not suited for that purpose today.

References

1. Campbell RWF. Atrial flutter. *Eur Heart J* 1998;19(suppl E):E37–E40.
2. Cox JL, Schuessler RB, Boineau JP. The surgical treatment of atrial fibrillation: I. Summary of the current concepts of the mechanisms of atrial flutter and atrial fibrillation. *J Thorac Cardiovasc Surg* 1991;101:402–405.
3. Ellis WS, SippensGroenewegen A, Lesh M. The effect of linear lesions on atrial defibrillation threshold and spontaneous termination–A computer modeling study. *Pacing Clinical Electrophysiol* 1997;20(II):1145. Abstract.

4. Cox JL, Schuessler RB, D'Agostino HJ, et al. The surgical treatment of atrial fibrillation: III. Development of a definite surgical procedure. *J Thorac Cardiovasc Surg* 1991;101:569–583.
5. Garg A, Finneran W, Mollerus M, et al. Right atrial compartmentalization using radiofrequency catheter ablation for management of patients with refractory atrial fibrillation. *J Cardiovasc Electrophysiol* 1999;10:763–771.
6. Kottkamp H, Hindricks G, Hammel D, et al. Intraoperative radiofrequency ablation of chronic atrial fibrillation: A left curative approach by elimination of anatomic "anchor" reentrant circuit. *J Cardiovasc Electrophysiol* 1999;10:772–780.
7. Haïssaguerre M, Jaïs P, Shah D, et al. Spontaneous initiation of atrial fibrillation by ectopic beats originating in the pulmonary veins. *N Engl J Med* 1998;339:659–666.

Chapter 17

Atrial Fibrillation:
A Clinician's Standpoint

Martin Fromer, MD

Introduction

Atrial fibrillation (AF) is the most frequent arrhythmia in patients over 65 years of age. Psaty et al. found an incidence of 19.2 per 1000 person-years, but it is by far not the most frequent arrhythmia that today's electrophysiologists deal with.[1] We all know that AF does harm to the patients. It has important impact on morbidity, mortality and health care consumption. Even if adjusted for age, hypertension, or myocardial infarction, etc., AF increases the risk of death by a factor 1.5.[2] Therefore, we would like to have an effective therapy, at best we would like to offer a cure for AF, but curative approaches need a definition of mechanisms.

What type of arrhythmia is AF really? Actually, one doubts whether anybody knows. Mapping studies have shown that AF has many faces and various types of AF have been described,[3,4] based on the degree of organization, number of wavelets and spatial distribution of wavelets. AF wavelets change over time in space, they split up and double, they are extinguished and unpredictable. But in dogs some anatomic areas were identified where unstable reentrant circuits are preferentially located.[5] How do those findings influence the treatment of patients? In humans identification of target areas are difficult. Could this be an application for computer simulation?

Today's antiarrhythmic drugs provide only nonspecific treatment. The exception may be adrenergically driven AF, that responds to beta-blockers. This type of AF is found after cardiovascular surgery, in conjunction with emotional or physical stress, or occurring mainly during

From Virag N, Blanc O, Kappenberger L (eds): *Computer Simulation and Experimental Assessment of Cardiac Electrophysiology.* ©Futura Publishing Co., Inc., Armonk, NY, 2001.

morning hours. Enhanced vagal tone may also lead to AF and drugs that have a vagolytic effect may be prescribed. Extensive ambulatory Holter recordings are used to document this rare type of AF.[6] Cardioversion by antiarrhythmic drugs, such as sotalol or amiodarone, has a limited efficacy and depends on the lapse of time after onset of AF, underlying heart disease, and left atrial dimension.[7–10] Associated with class 1 and 3 drugs is the risk to provoke QT-prolongation and polymorphic ventricular tachycardia.[11] A more electrophysiologic approach is electrical external cardioversion. How to prevent recurrence of AF after successful cardioversion? Again, antiarrhythmic drugs are prescribed, but recurrences are frequent.[10] Pacing of the atria in sick sinus syndrome may be indicated as well.

The finding of multiple wavelets with functional re-entry during AF has led to the concept of compartimentalization of the atria, the maze procedure that has been introduced by J. Cox.[12] Recently, various surgical teams have started to use radiofrequency (RF) current application endocardially and epicardially delivered by specially designed catheters.[13] Haïssaguerre et al. and others have replicated this by creating linear lesions in the atria using RF energy.[14,15] The observation that the right atrium may not be necessary for the perpetuation or initiation of AF, has led to interventions in the left atrium, with RF lesions encircling the pulmonary veins and going down to the mitral annulus.[16] The eagerness to be able to create continuous and transmural lesions to halt electrical conduction has driven the development of novel catheters and alternative energy sources to RF current.[17] However, nobody would actually pretend that prevention of persistent AF by catheter ablation has been achieved.

Clinical management of patients with AF has not only been influenced by the finding of multiple wavelets, but also by the observation that atrial fibrillation begets atrial fibrillation, that is, electrical remodelling during AF modifies the electrophysiologic characteristics of AF and perpetuates AF.[18] Translated to patient management, this means that repetitive cardioversion should prolong the AF-free intervals; on the other hand, prolonged recurrences of AF will lead to a more stable presentation of AF with transition to persistent AF. However, not all patients with repetitive paroxysms of AF really develop chronic AF. Repetitive cardioversion for recurrent AF is not always feasible. Implantable atrial cardioverters have not gained widespread use, mainly due to the pain associated with internal cardioversion and due to limitation in funding.

The therapeutic attitude towards persistent AF is generally pragmatic, as a cure seems actually almost impossible. The goal is to prevent complications: prevention of arterial emboli by effective anticoagulation and prevention of heart failure by prevention of rapid ventricular response. Catheter ablation of the atrio-ventricular junction has been shown to improve cardiac function in patients with tachycardic AF.[19]

APC

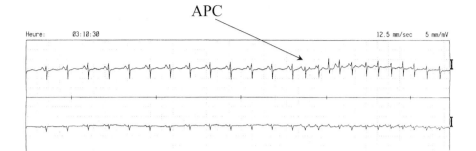

Figure 1. Induction of atrial tachycardia with transition to AF by a single APC (P on T), most likely originating from a pulmonary vein. Three years later the patient is in persistent AF.

The observation that atrial ectopic beats induce episodes of sustained AF has changed fundamentally the treatment strategies. Haïssaguerre et al. located by catheter mapping the origin of atrial ectopic beats within the first centimetres of the pulmonary veins (PV).[20] Muscle sleeves are responsible for the ectopic foci. The role of the muscle sleeves might be to

APC

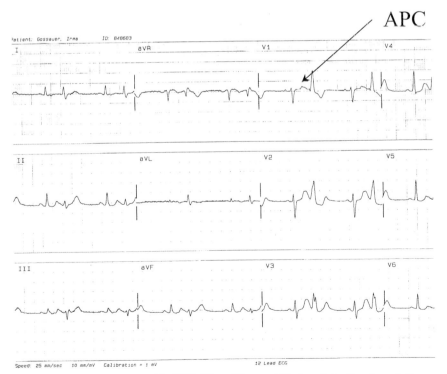

Figure 2. Atrial bigeminus with APC (P on T), most likely originating from left superior pulmonary vein. The patient has documented paroxysmal AF.

pump blood from the lungs to the left atrium. The same group found spike potentials (PV spikes) that are generated by these foci and selective mapping and ablation led to elimination of paroxysmal, recurrent AF.[21] Whether the spikes are due to micro-reentry or abnormal automaticity is not clear yet. The whole concept of AF management has been changed by the finding of these arrhythmogenic sources. Figure 1 shows an episode of AF initiation by a single atrial ectopic beat (atrial premature contraction, APC). Three years later the same patient presents with persistent AF. In Figure 2 an atrial bigeminus is documented originating from the left superior pulmonary vein (LSPV). The same patient also presents paroxysmal AF and underwent isolation of the pulmonary vein spikes by discrete RF ablation. Figure 3 shows the elimination of PV spikes by RF application. In Figure 4 a sequence of 2 short coupled PV spikes, interval 160 ms, is shown. The initiation of AF has been prevented in this case by amiodarone infusion. Figure 5 shows a mapping using a circular 10-polar catheter placed in the right superior PV. It shows the propagation of the spike potential within the vein that captures the atrial tissue and provokes a left atrial premature contraction. The pioneering work of Haissaguerre, Jais and Shah will modify, at least for a certain period of time, the man-

Paper speed 100 mm/s

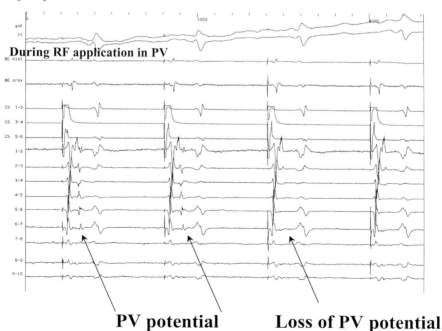

Figure 3. Elimination of PV spikes by RF application.

Paper speed 100 mm/s

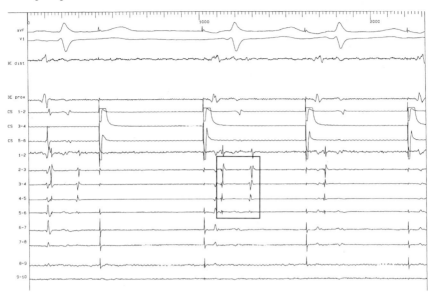

Figure 4. Double PV spike, 160 ms interval, dissociated from left atrium.

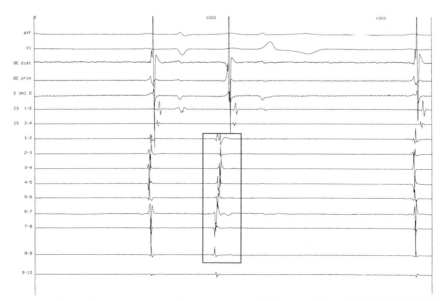

Figure 5. Recording of a propagation sequence of PV potentials. An atrial premature beat is initiated by this ectopic activity.

agement of AF patients. Questions arise such as: is lone persistent AF mainly the result of rapid firing foci with initially fibrillatory conduction in the atrial tissue that later, by electrical remodelling, transforms to persistent AF? Is it sufficient, although technically difficult at this state of technology, to isolate electric-anatomically the insertion of the pulmonary veins into the left atrium and to entrap the focus within the vein, for prevention of AF?

Anatomy is destiny, as has been said by Sigmund Freud, and the work of the clinical electrophysiologist is to modify the anatomy to prevent arrhythmia. Computer models may help to identify target zones improve understanding of mechanisms and help formulate concepts, but it is obviously extremely complex to model nature.

References

1. Psaty BM, Manolio TA, Kuller LH, et al. Incidence of and risk factors for atrial fibrillation in older adults. *Circulation* 1997;96:2455–2461.
2. Benjamin EJ, Wolf PA, D'Agostino RB, et al. Impact of atrial fibrillation on the risk of death. The Framingham Heart Study. *Circulation* 1998;98:946–952.
3. Allessie MA, Konings KTS. Mapping of atrial fibrillation in humans. In: Allessie MA, Fromer M. (eds). **Atrial and Ventricular Fibrillation: Mechanisms and Device Therapy**. Armonk, NY, Futura Publishing Company, 1997; 179–198.
4. Konings KTS, Smeets JLMR, Penn OC, et al. Configuration of unipolar atrial electrograms during electrically induced atrial fibrillation in humans. *Circulation* 1997;95:1231–1241.
5. Kumagai K, Khrestian C, Waldo AL. Simultaneous multisite studies during induced atrial fibrillation in the sterile pericarditis model. Insights into the mechanism of its maintenance. *Circulation* 1997;95:511–521.
6. Coumel P, Attuel P, Leclercq JF, et al. Arythmies auriculaires d'origine vagale ou catécholineregique. Effets comparés du traitment beta-bloquant et phénomène d'échappement. *Arch Mal Coeur* 1981;75:373–388.
7. Shenasa M, Kus T, Fromer M, et al. Effects of intravenous and oral calcium antagonists (Diltiazem and Verapamil) on sustenance of atrial fibrillation. *Am J Cardiol* 1988;62:403–407.
8. Van Gelder IC, Crijns HJGM, Van Gilst WH, et al. Efficacy and safety of flecainide acetate in the maintenance of sinus rhythm after electrical cardioversion of chronic atrial fibrillation or atrial flutter. *Am J Cardiol* 1989; 64:1317–1321.
9. Goy J, Métrailler J, Humair L, de Torrenté A. Restoration of sinus rhythm in atrial fibrillation of recent onset using intravenous propafenone. *Am Heart J* 1991;122:1788–1790.
10. Roy D, Talajic M, Dorian P, et al. Amiodarone to prevent recurrence of atrial fibrillation. *N Engl J Med* 2000;342:913–920.
11. Marcus FA. The hazards of using type 1C antiarrhythmic drugs for the treatment of paroxysmal atrial fibrillation. *Am J Cardiol* 1990;66:366–367.

12. Cox JL, Jaquiss RDB, Schuessler RB, et al. Modification of the Maze procedure for atrial fibrillation and atrial flutter. *J Thorac Cardiovasc Surg* 1995;110: 485–495.
13. Ruchat P, Schlaepfer J, Fromer M, et al. Traitement par radiofréquence de la fibrillation auriculaire chronique lors de la chirurgie mitrale. [Abstract] *Kardiovasculaer Medizin* 1999;2:71.
14. Haïssaguerre M, Marcus FI, Fischer B, et al. Radiofrequency catheter ablation in unusual mechanisms of atrial fibrillation: Report of three cases. *J Cardiovasc Electrophysiol* 1994;5:743–751.
15. Gaita F, Riccardi R, Calo L, et al. Atrial mapping and radiofrequency catheter ablation in patients with idiopathic atrial fibrillation. Electrophysiological findings and ablation results. *Circulation* 1998;97:2136–2145.
16. Pappone C, Rosanio S, Oreto G, et al. Circumferential radiofrequency ablation of pulmonary vein ostia. A new anatomic approach for curing atrial fibrillation. *Circulation* 2000;102:2619–2628.
17. Avitall B, Helms RW, Koblish JB, et al. The creation of linear contiguous lesions in the atria with an expandable loop catheter. *J Am Coll Cardiol* 1999;33:972–984.
18. Wijffels MCEF, Kirchhof CHHJ, Dorland R, et al. Atrial fibrillation begets atrial fibrillation. A study in awake chronically instrumented goats. *Circulation* 1995;92:1954–1968.
19. Brignole M, Menozzi C, Gianfranchi L, et al. Assessment of atrioventricular junction ablation and VVIR pacemaker versus pharmacological treatment in patients with heart failure and chronic atrial fibrillation - A randomized, controlled study. *Circulation* 1998:98: 953–960
20. Haïssaguerre M, Jaïs P, Shah DC, et al. Spontaneous initiation of atrial fibrillation by ectopic beats originating in the pulmonary veins. *N Engl J Med* 1998; 339:659–666.
21. Jais P, Haïssaguerre M, Shah DC, et al. A focal source of atrial fibrillation treated by discrete radiofrequency ablation. *Circulation* 1997;95:572–576.

Part VI.

Options in the Treatment of Ventricular Fibrillation

Chapter 18

Mechanisms of Ventricular Defibrillation

Nipon Chattipakorn, MD, PhD,
Raymond Ideker, MD, PhD

Introduction

Sudden cardiac death, mainly caused by ventricular fibrillation (VF), is responsible for over 250,000 deaths annually in the United States.[1] Currently, electrical defibrillation is the only practical means for terminating VF. The mortality rate from sudden cardiac death has decreased in the past decade, partly due to the improvement of our understanding of the nature of this fatality as well as the development of defibrillation devices. Recent advances in external defibrillators have led to the introduction of public access defibrillation, which promises to significantly reduce the mortality rate due to sudden cardiac death. Recent advances in implantable defibrillators, such as the use of a biphasic waveform, have led to smaller intravenous devices that have been shown to significantly benefit certain groups of patients.[2,3] Recent findings that post-shock activation always arises from the weakest shock field has led to the possible development of improved device therapy.[4,5] Despite these wide applications of transthoracic and intracardiac defibrillators, there is still a great need to improve defibrillation. In the past few decades, there have been advances in our understanding of the mechanism of defibrillation.[6-9] The better we understand the fundamental mechanisms of defibrillation, the more likely it is that we will be able to devise strategies to improve defibrillation.

[1] This work is supported in part by National Institutes of Health research grant HL-42760 and an award (0060295B) from the American Heart Association, Southeast Affiliate.

From Virag N, Blanc O, Kappenberger L (eds): *Computer Simulation and Experimental Assessment of Cardiac Electrophysiology.* ©Futura Publishing Co., Inc., Armonk, NY, 2001.

Effects of Shock Strengths on the Immediate Myocardial Responses to the Shock and the Post-Shock Activation Patterns: Is there one Mechanism for all Strength Shocks?

Although the mechanism of defibrillation has been investigated for many decades, it is still debated.[6–10] This is partly due to the fact that defibrillation is probabilistic and dependent on the shock strength.[11] Since the multi-channel electrical cardiac mapping technique was introduced, it has allowed investigators to record extracellular potentials from hundreds of sites on the ventricles simultaneously. Our understanding of how a shock succeeds or fails to defibrillate the heart has also rapidly progressed. A number of electrical cardiac mapping studies of defibrillation have demonstrated that following a near-defibrillation threshold (DFT) shock, there was a quiescent period when no electrical activity was observed, the so-called "isoelectric window."[12–15] Following this pause, the first post-shock activation usually arose in the region that was least affected by the shock, the weak shock potential gradient region, and then globally propagated across the entire myocardium.[14,15] This isoelectric window has been previously proposed to predict the outcome of defibrillation, i.e., successful defibrillation has a longer window than failed defibrillation.[12,13] Other studies, including optical mapping studies of defibrillation, which investigated the refractory period extension caused by the shock, also found that successful shocks cause longer refractory period extension than failed shocks.[16,17] It has been proposed that the extension of the refractory period caused by a successful shock over a critical mass of ventricular myocardium created less dispersion of refractoriness or a nearly uniform repolarization after the shock.[18] Thus, unidirectional propagated activation is unlikely to occur or to survive to generate a reentrant circuit that can bring the heart back into VF.[7,18] Shocks that fail to sufficiently prolong the refractoriness of myocardium will result in greater dispersion of refractoriness after the shock, allowing the initiation of reentry and VF to occur in failed defibrillation.[19,20] Although the importance of refractory period prolongation has been shown from electrical mapping studies, reentrant activation immediately following failed shocks near the DFT in strength is rarely observed. Following the near-DFT shocks, the first few post-shock activations often arose at the weak shock potential gradient region and focally propagated across the entire ventricles in an organized pattern before degenerating into VF in failed defibrillation episodes.[12–15] No reentry was observed immediately after the shock in these studies.

Recently, a new cardiac mapping technique that takes advantage of the ability of potentiometric dyes that bind to the cell membrane and change their fluorescence emission property with change in the transmembrane potential has been introduced to defibrillation research.[18,21,22] This optical mapping technique allows the investigators to directly observe both the depolarization and repolarization patterns of activation as well as cardiac responses during the shock, an interval that cannot be observed with electrical mapping studies. Reports from optical mapping studies, however, are somewhat inconsistent with electrical mapping studies. Optical mapping studies have found that there was no isoelectric window following the shock of the type reported from electrical mapping studies.[21,22] Instead, activation fronts were observed immediately after the shock, arising from either (a) the area that was directly excited by the shock and propagating into the less refractory area[21] or (b) the area of high transmembrane potential gradient between hyperpolarized and depolarized regions in which the activation front propagated from the depolarized into the hyperpolarized region.[22] This activation front then returned to the area that was refractory earlier but had now had time to recover by the time the activation front propagated through, forming a loop or a reentrant circuit.

This discrepancy has recently been studied and several solutions have been suggested to resolve these inconsistent results.[10,15] In the past decade, most electrical mapping studies have investigated the defibrillation mechanism using biphasic shocks of a strength near the DFT delivered to large-heart animal models, i.e., dogs and pigs.[12–15] Optical mapping studies, however, have investigated effects of defibrillation shocks by using monophasic shocks well below DFT strength delivered to isolated hearts of small animal models, i.e., guinea pigs or rabbits.[18,21,22] Are findings from one group right while the others are wrong? Probably not, since the experimental protocols are so different. But, to fully answer this question, an optical mapping study that uses various strength shocks (low- to high-voltage shocks) delivered to a fibrillating heart using a similar experimental set-up and study protocol as used in previous electrical mapping studies is needed. This study design will allow investigators to investigate whether 1) results from optical mapping or electrical mapping studies truly represent the defibrillation mechanism or 2) results from both groups are accurate but that optical mapping results demonstrate the effects of low strength shocks, whereas electrical mapping results represent the effects of near DFT strength shocks.

Post-Shock Activation Pattern after Failed Defibrillation of Near DFT Strength Shocks

Recent electrical mapping studies performed in open-chest pigs using only shocks near the DFT in strength have demonstrated that following near DFT shocks the characteristics of the first post-shock activation are not different between successful and failed shocks.[14,15] In failed defibrillation episodes, the first few activation fronts always arise rapidly and propagate slowly across the ventricles compared to the pattern seen in successful episodes (Figure 1).[14,15] A focal activation pattern was observed for the first few post-shock cycles before degenerating into VF in failed defibrillation episodes (Figure 2).[15] Reentry was not observed during the first few cycles after failed shocks in these studies. Because defibrillation is probabilistic and shock strength dependent, the inconsistencies of the results obtained from electrical and optical mapping studies could be caused by the different shock strengths used in those studies. To test this hypothesis, an optical mapping study which uses only near DFT shocks and performs in an experimental set-up and protocol similar to that of electrical mapping studies is needed. This has been achieved recently by Chattipakorn et al.[23–25] Their recent optical mapping studies performed in isolated pig hearts has demonstrated that following near DFT shocks, the

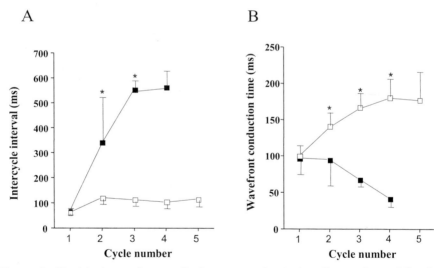

Figure 1. Electrical mapping results from open-chest pigs. Comparison of the first five post-shock cycles for shocks of equal strength near the DFT that either did (closed squares) or did not (open squares) defibrillate. Mean ± SD are shown for a total of 50 shocks in 5 pigs. There was no fifth ectopic cycle observed in any successful defibrillation episode. (A) The intercycle interval for cycle 1 is the time from the shock to the earliest recorded epicardial activation and for the other 4 cycles is the time between earliest activation for cycle N minus the time of earliest activation for cycle N-1. (B) Wavefront conduction time is the time for each activation cycle to propagate across the epicardium. It is the time interval from the earliest until the latest appearance of activation for that cycle. An asterisk indicates P<0.05 for that cycle for shocks that successfully defibrillated compared with those that failed to defibrillate. Cycle 1 is indistinguishable for successful and failed shocks by either measure. (Modified with permission from Chattipakorn et al.[15])

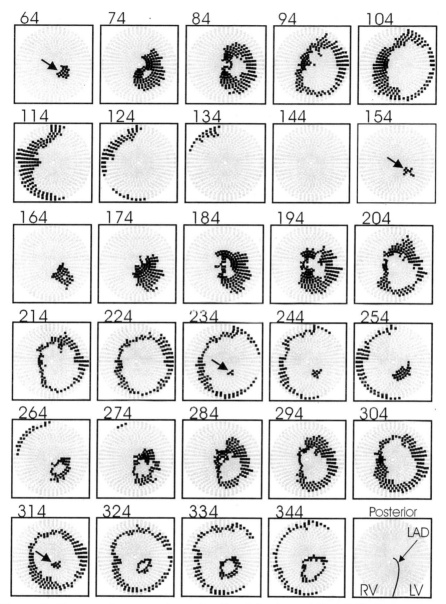

Figure 2. Frames of a computer animation following a failed defibrillation shock demonstrating the focal origin of the first four post-shock cycles in the lateral LV apex with organized propagation of these fronts across the epicardium. Each frame represents a polar view of the ventricular epicardium with the left anterior descending artery (LAD) represented by the long curved line at the bottom, the RV on the left and LV on the right with LV apex in the center. Numbers on top of each frame indicate the time from the shock. Consecutive frames are 10 ms apart. Each black dot represents activation at one of the 504 recording electrodes during that frame. Arrows indicate the early site for each cycle. These were the rapid cycles following a failed biphasic shock from electrodes in the RV apex and the SVC. (Modified with permission from Chattipakorn et al.[15])

159

first post-shock cycle is indistinguishable between successful and failed shocks. After failed defibrillation, the first few post-shock cycles always focally arise rapidly and propagate slowly, a similar pattern observed in electrical mapping studies.[23–25] No reentry was observed after the shock. They also demonstrated the existence of an isoelectric window after successful and failed shocks. Thus, results from both electrical and optical studies using shocks of near DFT strength consistently demonstrated that without the influence of shock strength, focal activation was the mechanism responsible for failed defibrillation.[14,15,23–25] These findings strongly suggest that previous observations of the relationship between the characteristics of the first post-shock cycle and shock outcome may be an effect of shock strength rather than a direct cause and effect relationship. Focal activation may be responsible for failed defibrillation for near-DFT strength shocks whereas reentry, which is rarely observed on the epicardium immediately after the near DFT shock for the first few post-shock activations, may be responsible for failed defibrillation when the shock strength is well below the DFT.[9,10]

Small Arrhythmogenic Region Following Near-DFT Shocks

Results from the near-threshold studies for both defibrillation[14,15] and VF induction[26] are all consistent in that, following the shock, the sites of earliest activation always arose at the left ventricular apex, the weak shock potential gradient region for the right ventricular (RV) apex-superior vena cava (SVC) shocking electrode configuration.[27] Activations arose repeatedly faster but in an organized pattern from this region for at least five cycles before degenerating into VF as observed in both defibrillation and VF induction studies.[14,15,26,28,29] It is not known what produces these post-shock activations and why this post-shock activity spontaneously stops after a few cycles leading to a successful defibrillation/failed VF induction in some cases, while it continues and generates VF leading to failed defibrillation/successful VF induction in others. However, these findings suggest the extreme importance of this small arrhythmogenic region after the shock. The similarity of the immediate post-shock activation pattern between successful and failed shocks suggests that the global dispersion of refractoriness following the shock may not be the key determinant for the success or failure of defibrillation in these normal hearts. Rather, the state of the small arrhythmogenic region from which the post-shock cycles arise is the crucial determinant of shock outcome.

Several recent studies strongly support this hypothesis. Studies in which a tiny shock, 50–100 V, was given to a small electrode on the epicardium at LV apex, the site of weakest potential gradient where the early post-shock cycles arise, just before or after the standard defibrillation shock was given from electrodes at the RV apex and SVC, have demonstrated that the total DFT energy was decreased by 60% compared with the DFT for shocks through the RV-SVC electrodes alone.[30–32] When the small electrode was placed elsewhere on the epicardium, it had little or no effect on the DFT. A recent VF induction study showed that the same general phenomenon occurred after the initiation of VF by a stimulus slightly larger than the VF threshold.[33] Defibrillation shocks delivered from an electrode immediately adjacent to the electrode from which VF was initiated could significantly lower the defibrillation threshold when shocks were delivered during the first three post-induction cycles compared with the defibrillation threshold for defibrillation shocks delivered after 10 seconds of VF, when activations no longer arose solely from the area of original initiation. In a recent study, subendocardial radiofrequency ablation was performed at the site where the early post-shock activation arose after VF induction by the near-threshold shocks.[34] Ablation of this arrhythmogenic region resulted in a marked decrease in the shock strength required not to induce VF, but when ablation was performed elsewhere, it had little or no effect on the this shock strength. All of these studies indicate the crucial importance of the small region that gives rise to activations after the shock in determining defibrillation outcome.

Despite the consistent findings from the near DFT shock studies from both electrical and optical mapping, one question remains unanswered, "Does intramural reentry exist?" It has been thought that focal activation observed in those near DFT defibrillation studies could be an epicardial breakthrough resulting from intramural reentry which could not be detected due to the limitation of the epicardial mapping technique. Future 3-D mapping is necessary to answer this question.

References

1. Zipes DP, Wellens HJJ. Sudden cardiac death. *Circulation* 1998;98:2334–2351.
2. Zipes DP, Roberts D. Results of the international study of the implantable pacemaker cardioverter-defibrillator: A comparison of epicardial and endocardial lead systems. *Circulation* 1995;92:59–65.
3. Maron BJ, Shen WK, Link MS, et al. Efficacy of implantable cardioverter-defibrillators for the prevention of sudden death in patients with hypertrophic cardiomyopathy. *N Engl J Med* 2000;342:365–373.
4. Meisel E, Butter C, Philippon F, et al. Transvenous biventricular defibrillation. *Am J Cardiol* 2000;86:K76-K85.
5. Roberts PR, Urban JF, Euler DE, et al. The middle cardiac vein—a novel pathway to reduce the defibrillation threshold. *J Interv Card Electrophysiol* 1999; 3:55–60.

6. Chen PS, Swerdlow CD, Hwang C, et al. Current concepts of ventricular defibrillation. *J Cardiovasc Electrophysiol* 1998;9:553–562.

7. Dillon SM, Kwaku KF. Progressive depolarization: A unified hypothesis for defibrillation and fibrillation induction by shocks. *J Cardiovasc Electrophysiol* 1998;9:529–52.

8. Efimov IR, Gray RA, Roth BJ. Virtual electrodes and deexcitation: New insights into fibrillation induction and defibrillation. *J Cardiovasc Electrophysiol* 2000;11:339–353.

9. Chattipakorn N, Ideker RE. Mechanism of Defibrillation. In: Aliot E, Clémenty J, Prystowsky EN (eds). **Fighting Sudden Cardiac Death: A Worldwide Challenge**. Armonk, NY, Futura Publishing Co.: 2000:593–615.

10. Ideker RE, Chattipakorn N, Gray RA. Defibrillation Mechanisms: The Parable of the Blind Men and the Elephant? *J Cardiovasc Electrophysiol* 2000;11: 1008–1013.

11. Davy JM, Fain ES, Dorian P, et al. The relationship between successful defibrillation and delivered energy in open-chest dogs: Reappraisal of the "defibrillation threshold" concept. *Am Heart J* 1987;113:77–84.

12. Chen P-S, Shibata N, Dixon EG, et al. Activation during ventricular defibrillation in open-chest dogs: Evidence of complete cessation and regeneration of ventricular fibrillation after unsuccessful shocks. *J Clin Invest* 1986;77: 810–823.

13. Shibata N, Chen P-S, Dixon EG, et al. Epicardial activation following unsuccessful defibrillation shocks in dogs. *Am J Physiol* 1988;255:H902-H909.

14. Usui M, Callihan RL, Walker RG, et al. Epicardial sock mapping following monophasic and biphasic shocks of equal voltage with an endocardial lead system. *J Cardiovasc Electrophysiol* 1996;7:322–334.

15. Chattipakorn N, Fotuhi PC, Ideker RE. Prediction of defibrillation outcome by epicardial activation patterns following shocks near the defibrillation threshold. *J Cardiovasc Electrophysiol* 2000;11:1014–1021.

16. Sweeney RJ, Gill RM, Steinberg MI, et al. Ventricular refractory period extension caused by defibrillation shocks. *Circulation* 1990;82:965–972.

17. Tovar OH, Jones JL. Relationship between "extension of refractoriness" and probability of successful defibrillation. *Am J Physiol* 1997;272:H1011-H1019.

18. Dillon SM. Synchronized repolarization after defibrillation shocks: A possible component of the defibrillation process demonstrated by optical recordings in rabbit heart. *Circulation* 1992;85:1865–1878.

19. Jones JL, Tovar OH. The mechanism of defibrillation and cardioversion. *Proc IEEE* 1996;84:392–403.

20. Frazier DW, Wolf PD, Wharton JM, et al. Stimulus-induced critical point: Mechanism for electrical initiation of reentry in normal canine myocardium. *J Clin Invest* 1989;83:1039–1052.

21. Kwaku KF, Dillon SM. Shock-induced depolarization of refractory myocardium prevents wave-front propagation in defibrillation. *Circ Res* 1996;79:957–973.

22. Efimov IR, Cheng Y, Van Wagoner DR, et al. Virtual electrode-induced phase singularity: A basic mechanism of defibrillation failure. *Circ Res* 1998;82: 918–925.

23. Chattipakorn N, Banville I, Gray RA, et al. Mechanism of ventricular defibrillation for near-defibrillation-threshold shocks: A whole heart optical mapping study in swine. *Circulation* 2000;102:II-340.
24. Chattipakorn N, Banville I, Gray RA, et al. Regional myocardial response to defibrillation shocks is a key determinant for shock outcome: An optical mapping study in swine. *J Am Coll Cardiol* 2001 (in press).
25. Chattipakorn N, Banville I, Gray RA, et al. Mechanisms of VF reinitiation after failed defibrillation shocks: An optical mapping study in isolated swine hearts. *J Am Coll Cardiol* 2001. In Press.
26. Chattipakorn N, Rogers JM, Ideker RE. Influence of postshock epicardial activation patterns on initiation of ventricular fibrillation by upper limit of vulnerability shocks. *Circulation* 2000;101:1329–1336.
27. Tang ASL, Wolf PD, Claydon FJ, et al. Measurement of defibrillation shock potential distributions and activation sequences of the heart in three-dimensions. *Proc IEEE* 1988;76:1176–1186.
28. Chattipakorn N, Fotuhi PC, Sreenan KM, et al. Pacing after shocks stronger than the upper limit of vulnerability: Impact on fibrillation induction. *Circulation* 2000;101:1337–1343.
29. Chattipakorn N, Fotuhi PC, Ideker RE. Pacing following shocks stronger than the defibrillation threshold: Impact on defibrillation outcome. *J Cardiovasc Electrophysiol* 2000;11:1022–1028.
30. Walker RG, KenKnight BH, Ideker RE. Impact of low-amplitude auxiliary shock strength on endocardial defibrillation threshold reductions with novel dual-shock therapy. *Pacing Clin Electrophysiol* 1998;21:900.
31. Walker RG, KenKnight BH, Ideker RE. Reduction of defibrillation threshold by 50% with a low-amplitude auxiliary shock. *Pacing Clin Electrophysiol* 1998;21:853.
32. KenKnight BH, Walker RG, Ideker RE. Marked reduction of ventricular defibrillation threshold by application of an auxiliary shock to a catheter electrode in the left posterior coronary vein of dogs [In Process Citation]. *J Cardiovasc Electrophysiol* 2000;11:900–906.
33. Strobel JS, Kenknight BH, Rollins DL, et al. The effects of ventricular fibrillation duration and site of initiation on the defibrillation threshold during early ventricular fibrillation. *J Am Coll Cardiol* 1998;32:521–7.
34. Chattipakorn N, Fotuhi PC, Zheng X, et al. Left ventricular apex ablation decreases the upper limit of vulnerability. *Circulation* 2000;101:2458–2460.

Chapter 19

Induction of Reentry and Defibrillation:

The Role of Virtual Electrodes

Natalia Trayanova, PhD

Introduction to the Concepts of Reentry Induction and Defibrillation

For a defibrillation shock to be successful, first the shock must extinguish existing activation fronts throughout the myocardium, and second, the shock must not initiate new reentrant activations. Thus, to understand defibrillation, we must understand (1) how propagation of pre-existing activity is prevented by the shock, and (2) how the shock induces reentry (i.e., shock-induced arrhythmogenesis). The critical point hypothesis for reentry induction introduced by Wiggers & Wegria[1] and expanded by Winfree[2] centers around the idea that an electrical shock generates an extracellular potential gradient[3] that falls off with the distance from the shock electrode. Experimental results of electrically recorded post-shock transmembrane potential behavior are consistent with this hypothesis.[3-5] Suppose that the electrical shock (S2) is delivered prematurely to a propagating action potential wave (elicited by a brief stimulus S1 from a location other than the location of the S2 shock). The intersection of a critical extracellular potential gradient isoline and a critical recovery isoline of this propagating wave is the 'critical point' around which a rotor will be formed.[2] The rotor ensues because the S2 extracellular potential gradient correlates directly with the induced transmembrane potential;[6] the rise in

[1] Supported by NSF grants BES-9809132 and DMF-9709754, NIH grant HL63195, and by a contract LEQSF(1998–01)-RD-A-30 from the Louisiana Board of Regents through the Board of Regents Support Fund.

From Virag N, Blanc O, Kappenberger L (eds): *Computer Simulation and Experimental Assessment of Cardiac Electrophysiology.* ©Futura Publishing Co., Inc., Armonk, NY, 2001.

transmembrane potential in the wake of a propagating wavefront creates a unidirectional block and thus, conditions for reentrant activity.

As long as the critical point remains within the boundaries of the myocardium, the tissue is vulnerable to reentry. The 'upper limit of vulnerability' (ULV) is reached when the shock is so strong that the critical potential gradient isoline is at or beyond the borders of the myocardium. Above the ULV, an electric shock cannot initiate reentry. Thus, a successful defibrillation shock has to not only prevent propagation of pre-existing activity, but has to be above the ULV so it will not initiate new reentrant activations.[7]

How does the electric shock prevent the propagation of pre-existing fibrillatory activations? The key concept is the presumed direct relationship between extracellular potential gradient and shock-induced transmembrane potential mentioned above. Any portion of the tissue exposed to a significant extracellular potential gradient, determined experimentally to be above 5 V/cm,[8] will respond with a rise in the transmembrane potential. Shock-induced depolarization of a region undergoing fibrillatory activity translates into (1) activation of the pre-shock excitable gap, and (2) extension of local refractoriness for cells undergoing activation (graded response). Therefore, the majority of tissue becomes refractory and pre-existing reentrant wavefronts die out since they have nowhere to go.[9] Arrhythmia is obliterated and the defibrillation shock succeeds.

Virtual Electrode Polarization

The mechanisms presented above were conjectured from experimental recordings of electrical activity following the defibrillation shock. Overwhelming electrical artifacts prevented researchers from recording during as well as shortly after the shock. The breakthrough in mapping cardiac activity associated with defibrillation occurred with the introduction of potentiometric dyes, allowing observation of electrical activity in the heart during electric shocks. Simultaneously, bidomain simulations demonstrated the presence of oppositely polarized shock-induced areas throughout the myocardium, as if produced by 'virtual electrodes' (see reviews by Trayanova[10] and Efimov[11]). Further, the shock-induced transmembrane potential was not found to be directly related to the extracellular potential gradient.[12] Optical mapping studies[12–15] convincingly confirmed these theoretical predictions. It also became clear that both the external field and the tissue structure are major determinants of the shape, location, polarity and intensity of the virtual electrode polarization (VEP).[10,16]

The shock-induced hyperpolarization is the key element in the new understanding of defibrillation since it affects the pre-shock electrical activity in the heart. To understand that, one needs to consider what is the effect of shock-induced hyperpolarization on action potentials. The action potential duration can be either extended or shortened by either shock polarity depending on shock strength and coupling interval. However, the greatest effect is the complete de-excitation of the membrane (quick return to rest) caused by the hyperpolarizing effect of the shock. The fact that strong shock-induced hyperpolarization can abolish the action potential means that a new excitable gap can be created during the shock. For very strong shocks, this excitable gap depends only on the shape and location of the virtual anodes in the myocardium and is no longer a function of pre-shock activity.[11] Overall, pre-existing activity and shock-induced depolarization and hyperpolarization combine to create a post-shock distribution of transmembrane potential: certain regions are depolarized while excitability is restored in others. The outcome of the shock depends on this post-shock activity, but more importantly, on the interaction between the oppositely polarized areas.

The close proximity of a virtual anode and a virtual cathode can result in a break excitation at the end of the shock.[17] The depolarization of a virtual cathode serves as a electrical stimulus eliciting a propagating wave in the newly recovered virtual anode. The new activations arise at the borders between oppositely polarized areas provided that the gradient of polarization at the site of origin is sufficient to elicit an action potential.[18] The larger the gradient at the borders between oppositely polarized areas, the smaller the post-shock latency of the break excitations.[19] The propagation velocity of the break excitation through the post-shock excitable gaps depends on the level of the negative polarization: the more hyperpolarized a virtual anode is, the faster a break wavefront will propagate through it.[18] Often, the break excitations combine with remnants of pre-shock activity to form the post-shock waveforms.[19]

When do the post-shock wavefronts result in reentry? The survival of the break excitations depends, ultimately, on the strength of the shock. In the negatively polarized areas, the stronger shock elicits break excitations earlier after the end of the shock, and in greater numbers;[19] these also propagate faster. Thus, the post-shock activations will traverse the post-shock excitable gap more quickly and arrive at the border with the virtual cathode(s) earlier, before this area has recovered from refractoriness. In addition, in the areas of shock-induced depolarization, the stronger shock extends refractoriness more. Therefore, the stronger shock 'ensures' that propagation of post-shock activations through post-shock excitable gaps is terminated by their encounter with regions of extended refractoriness.

Figure 1 illustrates two examples of reentry induction by the shock. The top panels in the figure illustrate the pre-shock state of the tissue for each pair of simulations. Columns A and B show examples of a shock delivered at a coupling interval of 90ms; shock strength is 30 and 90 A/m^3,

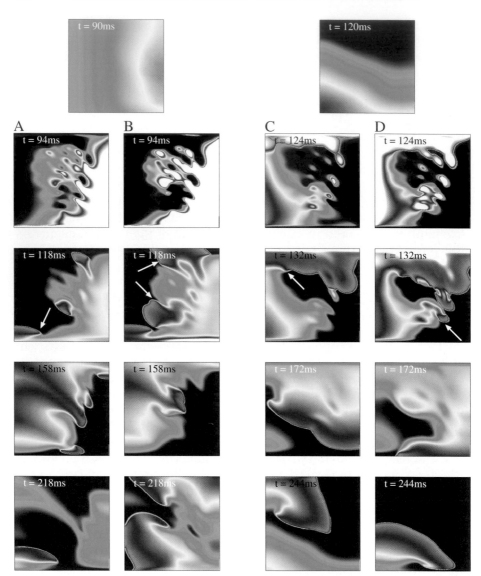

Figure 1. Post-shock wavefront dynamics in two pairs of simulations. Top panels show pre-shock activity. The shock is delivered via a line electrode at the horizontal top tissue border: A and B - cathodal cross-filed stimulation at a coupling interval of 90 ms; C and D - anodal parallel-field stimulation at a coupling interval of 120 ms. Shock strengths are 30 (A), 90 (B), -20 (C), and -50A/m^3 (D). Color scheme ranges between black (-100 mV) and white (50 mV); potentials outside the range are presented as black and white. Blue represents potentials around rest, red corresponds to depolarization associated with the propagated action potential, and other colors represent polarization linearly within this transmembrane potential range.

respectively. Comparting the t=94ms panels, the polarization pattern generated by the shock is much stronger in column B. As a result, more break wavefronts occur in column B and propagation through deexcited regions progresses faster. For the break wavefront near the center of the t=118ms panels, the propagation speed increases from 28 cm/s in column A to 51cm/s in column B. The upper break wavefronts shown in the t=118ms panels exhibit a similar increase in conduction velocity, from 27cm/s in column A to 41cm/s in column B. Further, comparing the same panels, one notices that the depolarization in the central portion of the tissue lingers longer in column B than in column A, demonstrating that the stronger shock results in a greater extension of refractoriness. Individual white arrows in the same panels indicate the wavefronts which ultimately lead to reentry in each simulation. Similar phenomena are observed in columns C and D.

Clearly, the effect of the defibrillation shock is not only in its depolarization of cardiac membranes, but in the creation of a new post-shock excitable gap. The success of a defibrillation episode lies with the successful eradication of this excitable gap before the adjacent regions recover from refractoriness. A failed defibrillation episode is associated with a slower propagation of the post-shock wavefronts through the excitable gap providing ample time for the adjacent depolarization to recede and open a pathway for further propagation.

VEP and the Critical Point Hypothesis

The VEP hypothesis for defibrillation makes little distinction between terminating pre-existing wavefronts and not re-initiating reentry. The alternative concept of defibrillation views success as (1) depolarization as means of prevention of propagation and (2) ensuring the critical point is outside the borders of the myocardium. Thus, in areas of high extracellular potential gradient the pre-existing wavefronts are terminated, while in low-gradient areas a critical point is formed and a new reentry ensues. In contrast, the VEP hypothesis is concerned only with the post-shock distribution of transmembrane potential, and more specifically, with the speedy eradication of post-shock excitable gap by post-shock wavefronts in advance of the recovery of the adjacent depolarized areas. If the post-shock excitable gap is not erased in time, defibrillation fails. Clearly, these concepts also apply to initiation of reentry by the shock. Indeed, if the shock is delivered during sinus rhythm and the post-shock excitable gap is not quickly eradicated, reentry ensues; the tissue is then in the vulnerable window. The ULV is reached when wavefronts propagating through the post-shock excitable gap reach refractory tissue and die out.

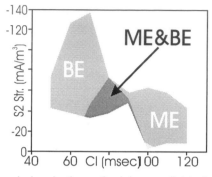

Figure 2. Vulnerability window in the cathodal cross-field stimulation protocol. See text for details.

The challenge facing researchers in defibrillation now is to reconcile the new understanding of the mechanisms for defibrillation with the existing electrical-recording experimental evidence[3–5] supporting the critical point hypothesis. A simulation study of ours[20] made one of the first attempts in this direction. It examined the vulnerability window for various stimulation protocols. Figure 2 illustrates the window of vulnerability as a function of coupling interval (CI) and S2 strength for cathodal cross-field stimulation (as in Figures 1 A and B) since the experimental studies supporting the critical point hypothesis were conducted for the same stimulation protocol (the critical point hypothesis does not predict reentry in the case of anodal shocks). In the regions labeled BE and ME in Figure 2, a single spiral wave is generated by either break or make excitation, respectively. The region labeled BE & ME represents a transition from break to make where both types of excitation give rise to figure of eight reentry. The S2 strength required to initiate reentry is greater for break than make excitation. The experimental studies supporting the critical point hypothesis[3–5] were conducted at long coupling intervals and below the S2 strengths required for break excitation which corresponds to the ME region on the graph. The distinct separation of the vulnerable window into two parts explains why these studies have missed the vulnerable window at short CIs. Our study demonstrates that the VEP hypothesis is consistent with the critical point hypothesis and experimental observation in the ME region, but not in the BE and BE & ME regions. Thus, the VEP theory of vulnerability encompasses the critical point hypothesis for cathodal shocks at long CIs while extending our understanding of the mechanisms of reentry induction and defibrillation to include the polarization by the shock and break excitation phenomena.

References

1. Wiggers CJ, Wegria R. Ventricular fibrillation due to single localized induction in condenser shock supplied during the vulnerable phase of the ventricular systole. *Am J Physiol* 1939;128:500–505.
2. Winfree AT. When time breaks down, *Princeton UP*, 1997.
3. Frazier DW, Wolf PD, Wharton J, et al. Stimulus-induced critical point: Mechanism electrical initiation of reentry in normal canine myocardium. *J Clin Invest* 1989;83:1039–1052.
4. Gotoh M, Uchida T, Mandel WJ, et al. Cellular graded responses and ventricular vulnerability to reentry by a premature stimulus in isolated canine ventricle. *Circulation* 1997;95:2141–2154.
5. Shibata N, Chen P-S, Dixon E, et al. Influence of shock strength and timing on induction of ventricular arrhythmias in dogs. *Am J Physiol* 1988;255:H891-H901.
6. Krassowska W, Pilkington TC, Ideker RE. The closed form solution to the periodic core-conductor model using asymptotic analysis. *IEEE Trans Biomed Eng* 1987;34:519–531.
7. Chen P-S, Shibata N, Dixon E, et al. Activation during ventricular defibrillation in open-chest dogs: Evidence of complete cessation and regeneration of ventricular fibrillation after unsuccessful shocks. *J Clin Invest* 1986;77:810–823.
8. Ideker RE, Wolf PD, Tang A. Mechanisms of defibrillation. In Tacker WA (ed): **Defibrillation of the Heart**, St. Louis, MO, Mosby Year Book, 1994, pp. 15–45.
9. Sweeney RJ, Gill RM, Reid PR. Characterization of refractory period extension by transcardiac shock. *Circulation* 1991;83:2057–2066.
10. Trayanova NA, Skouibine K, Aguel F. The role of cardiac tissue structure in defibrillation. *Chaos* 1998;8:221–233.
11. Efimov IR, Gray RA, Roth BJ. Virtual electrodes and de-excitation: New insights into fibrillation induction and defibrillation. *J Cardiovasc Electrophysiol* 2000;11:339–353.
12. Knisley SB, Blitchington TF, Hill BC, et al. Optical measurements of transmembrane potential changes during electrical field stimulation of ventricular cells. *Circ Res* 1993;72:255–270.
13. Efimov I, Cheng YN, Biermann M, et al. Transmembrane voltage changes produced by real and virtual electrodes during monophasic defibrillation shock delivered by an implantable electrode. *J Cardiovasc Electrophys* 1997;8:1031–1045.
14. Knisley SB, Trayanova NA, Aguel F. Roles of electric field and fibre structure in cardiac electric stimulation. *Biophys J* 1999;77:1404–1417.
15. Wikswo JP Jr, Lin SF, Abbas RA. Virtual electrodes in cardiac tissue: A common mechanism for anodal and cathodal stimulation. *Biophys J* 1995;69:2195–2210.
16. Sobie EA, Susil RC, Tung L. A generalized activating function for predicting virtual electrodes in cardiac tissue. *Biophys J* 1997;73:1410–1423.

17. Roth BJ. A mathematical model of make and break electrical stimulation of cardiac tissue by a unipolar anode or cathode. *IEEE Trans Biomed Eng* 1995;42:1174–1184.

18. Cheng Y, Mowrey KA, Van Wagoner DR, et al. Virtual electrode induced re-excitation: A mechanism of defibrillation. *Circ Res* 1999;85:1056–1066.

19. Skouibine K, Trayanova NA, Moore P. Success and failure of the defibrillation shock: Insights from a simulation study. *J Cardiovasc Electrophysiol* 2000;11: 785–796.

20. Lindblom A, Trayanova NA, Aguel F. Vulnerability to far-field stimulation: Virtual electrode polarization and critical point hypothesis. *J Cardiovasc Electrophysiol* 2000 (in review).

Chapter 20

Virtual Electrode Hypothesis of Stimulation of the Heart

Igor R. Efimov, PhD

Introduction

The ability of electric current to stimulate nerves and muscles was firmly established in 18th century.[1,2] Researchers of the 19th century discovered that an electric stimulus can induce cardiac arrest[3,4] or stop the arrhythmia.[5] Yet, it took another century of research to take a clinical advantage of the electric stimulation in the form of clinical pacing[6] and defibrillation.[7] Now, in the beginning of 21st century we are able to correct numerous heart rhythm abnormalities by electronic devices, which are based on principles of stimulation.

Despite impressive clinical success of both pacing and defibrillation, basic mechanisms of these phenomena remain unclear. Many generations of brilliant scientists tried to resolve this old puzzle.[8] Yet, until recently all these attempts were hampered by the inability of conventional electrode recording techniques to reproduce a behavior of cardiac cells during electric stimuli. Electric stimulus always resulted in a large artifact overwhelming a minute cellular response. Advent of optical means to measure transmembrane voltage made a world of difference in this area of research.[9] This method is based on a custom-designed spectroscopic properties of so-called voltage-sensitive dyes,[10] which respond by a spectral shift or intensity change to a change in transmembrane voltage. Finally, this method enabled researchers to visualize electrical activity during stimulus application.

The theory predicted that an extracellularly applied stimulus produces a biphasic effect on excitable membrane of nerves[11] or cardiac syncitium,[12] consisting of a simultaneous occurrence of positive and neg-

From Virag N, Blanc O, Kappenberger L (eds): *Computer Simulation and Experimental Assessment of Cardiac Electrophysiology.* ©Futura Publishing Co., Inc., Armonk, NY, 2001.

ative polarization of the membrane in adjacent regions. These opposite polarizations were considered to be driven by virtual sources, known as activating function[11,13] or virtual electrodes.[14] In the latter case, positive and negative polarizations are considered to be driven by virtual cathode and virtual anode, respectively.[14] Studies of virtual electrode polarization (VEP) resulted in formulation of virtual electrode theory of stimulation/defibrillation.[15]

In our studies, we used Langendorff-perfused rabbit hearts, which were stained with voltage-sensitive dye di-4-ANEPPS.[16] Electrical activity was monitored with a 16×16 photodiode array (Hamamatsu, Japan) at a rate of 1000–3000 frames/second. Depending on the task the field of view was adjusted from 4×4 to 20×20 mm. We studied three *in vitro* models of clinical stimulation/defibrillation of the heart: (1) *pacing* with unipolar and bipolar electrodes placed at the epicardium, (2) *ICD defibrillation* with a right ventricular electrode, and (3) *external defibrillation* with a pair of mesh electrodes positioned at both sides from the heart.

Mechanisms of Pacing

Using voltage-sensitive dyes several groups have presented evidence of VEP during unipolar epicardial stimulation,[14,17,18] which takes on a so-called "dog-bone" shape[12] near the stimulating electrode and the two oppositely polarized regions at both sides. Wikswo et al. presented a theory that explains both make and break stimulation, based on VEP.

We investigated VEP during both unipolar and bipolar 2-msec anodal and cathodal monophasic stimulation applied during diastole. Stimulus intensity varied from 10 μA to 40 mA. In agreement with previous findings we observed the "dog-bone" polarization produced by unipolar stimulation (see upper panels in Figure 1). Bipolar stimulation (lower panels of Figure 1) produced more complex VEP patterns, which represent superimposition of two unipolar patterns.[19]

Surprisingly, we have observed two different patterns of the origin of the heartbeat depending on the strength of the stimulus. Wikswo et al.[14] demonstrated that during make stimulation, the heartbeat originates from areas of the virtual cathode, which depolarized the tissue. In contrast, during break stimulation, the heartbeat originated from the areas of virtual anode, which hyperpolarized the tissue.[14] In fact, the latter was termed "break-excitation" because it was considered possible only during break-stimulation.

Our findings disagreed. We did observe a characteristic Wikswo's make stimulation, with the heartbeat originating at depolarized areas (not shown). But only with a strong stimuli amplitude of which exceeded 3–4 times the threshold value. In contrast (see Figure 2), weaker

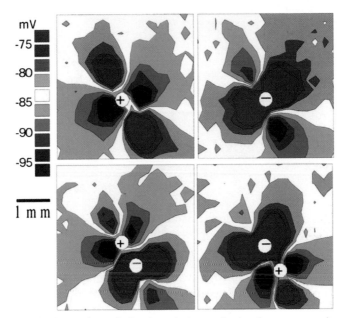

Figure 1. Virtual electrode polarization during unipolar (upper maps) and bipolar stimulation (lower maps). Square pulses 2-msec in duration and both polarities were applied during diastole. Transmembrane voltage was measured using optical mapping techniques. Maps show transmembrane voltage distribution 1-msec after the onset of the stimulus.

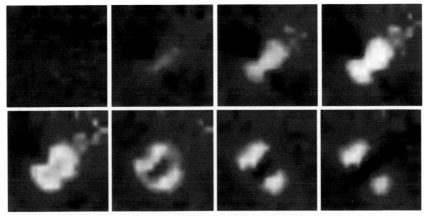

Figure 2. Origin of the heartbeat during unipolar cathodal make stimulation. Maps show distribution of first derivatives of the transmembrane potential (dV/dt) during and after the 2-msec pulse. Maps were measured 528 μsec apart. Notice (lower-left map), that the wavefront survives only in the initially hyperpolarized region.

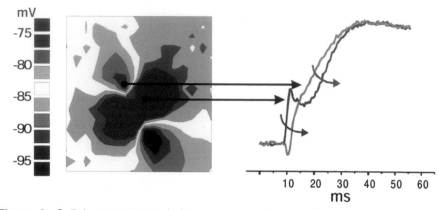

Figure 3. Cellular responses during paradoxical "break"-like heartbeat origin produced by make stimulation. Field of view is 4 × 4 mm. See text for detail.

near threshold stimuli induced a heartbeat originating at the hyperpolarized regions, as it would be expected during break stimulation. Figure 3 shows cellular responses from the areas of virtual anode and virtual cathode. These responses illustrate that initial depolarization by virtual cathode was insufficient to produce full response. Yet, hyperpolarization resulted in supernormal excitability in the area of virtual anode. This supernormal excitability was utilized by the driving force from incompletely depolarized areas of virtual cathode (red arrow) and resulted in overshooting of the resting potential value and full depolarization, which then provided driving force to areas of incomplete depolarization (blue arrow).

Thus, we conclude, that both modes of wavefront generation are observed during make excitation, depending on the stimulus strength.

Mechanisms of ICD Defibrillation

ICD defibrillation was modeled by a shock application from a 1-cm electrode inserted into the right ventricular cavity of a rabbit heart (see Figure 4). Monophasic and biphasic shocks of both polarities, ±50–260-V amplitude and 8-msec duration were applied during normal rhythm and during arrhythmia, produced by T-wave shocks. Measurements of the transmembrane voltage were conducted from the epicardium.

We observed VEP, which unlike pacing-induced patterns occupied an entire heart. Defibrillation shock induced VEP is supposed to produce an effect on fibrillating myocardium, which is in various phases of electrical activity prior to the shock application. Therefore, we investigated effect of VEP on refractory myocardium. We found that shocks applied during refractory periods produced three types of responses (see Figure 4): (1) de-excitation, (2) APD prolongation, and (3) re-excitation. Positive polarization results in an extension of the action potential duration and refractory period. Let us assign a value on a phase of electrical activity ranging from 0 to 2π when a cell undergoes changes from the upstroke to full recovery. In this case positive polarization (see red traces in Figure 4) resulted in a reduction of the pre-shock phase ϕ of electrical activity, $\phi' = \phi - \Delta$. This reduction is a monotonic function of positive polarization. Yet, the phase cannot be less than 0. In contrast, negative polarization is capable to result in a "jump" of phase by a complete cycle of 2π. Indeed, if a negative polarization is of moderate amplitude (blue traces), de-excitation[20] is observed. De-excitation results in an abbreviation of the action potential duration and refractory period. Moderate de-excitation (blue trace) does not restore excitability. It simply increases the pre-shock phase ϕ by some Δ, $\phi' = \phi + \Delta$. If negative polarization is strong enough, calcium and sodium channels reach the recovery from inactivation and the cells become excitable. Due to the proximity of the positively polarized region a strong gradient of transmembrane voltage develops at the boundary between the positively and negatively polarized regions. Such a gradient results in break-excitation, which forms a new wavefront,

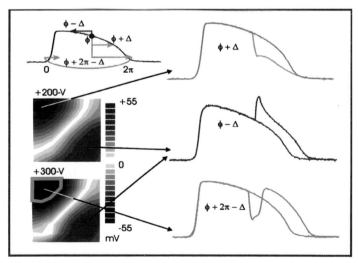

Figure 4. Optical recordings of three types of responses produced by virtual electrode polarization applied to refractory tissue. Weak negative polarization (right blue traces) shortens action potential duration and refractory period, advancing the phase (see the upper-left panel). Positive polarization (red traces) extends action potential duration, reducing the phase. Strong negative polarization (green traces) de-excites the tissue, restoring excitability and creating conditions from post-shock break-excitation. This advances the phase by more than a whole period (2π).

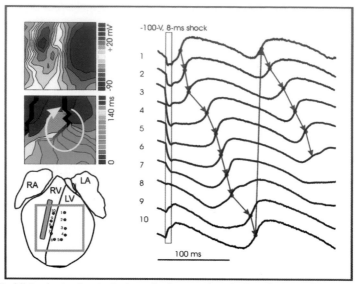

Figure 5. Virtual electrode induced phase singularity during ICD defibrillation. Monophasic, 100-V, 8-msec cathodal shock was applied in an attempt to arrest ventricular tachycardia. Shock produced characteristic VEP pattern (the upper-left panel), which terminated arrhythmic pattern. Yet, it resulted in a shock-induced phase singularity, which caused a new reentry (the middle left panel). Optical signals on the right panel show responses recorded around the phase singularity (along the reentrant circuit). Location of the recording sites is shown in the lower-left panel. Field of view is 18 × 18 mm.

re-exciting de-excited region. Thus, pre-shock phase f undergoes a jump exceeding 2π, $\phi' = \phi + 2\pi - \Delta$. This "jump" creates conditions for the development of a phase singularity, which is known to be a necessary condition for inducing a vortex-like source of electrical activity, also known as reentry. Figure 5 illustrates such a phenomenon, virtual electrode induced phase singularity, which was produced by a monophasic shock, applied in order to extinguish the arrhythmia. Shock succeeded in extinguishing the pre-shock arrhythmia. Yet, it re-induced a new arrhythmia, which caused the failure of defibrillation.[21]

Thus, we conclude that internal defibrillation monophasic shocks produce large-scale VEP, which may result in virtual electrode induced phase singularities, responsible for defibrillation failure. Our results also demonstrated that during biphasic shocks, the first phase induces virtual electrode induced phase singularity, while the second phase extinguishes them, eliminating the danger of re-inducing the arrhythmia. This explains superiority of biphasic shocks over monophasic ones.[21]

Mechanisms of External Defibrillation

External defibrillation was simulated *in vitro* by applying electric shocks from a pair of mesh electrodes positioned at both sides from the heart.[16] Optical mapping revealed VEP (see Figure 6). Yet, myocardial polarization during external defibrillation is driven by different structural mechanisms. In order to explore these mechanisms, Felipe Aguel used an anatomically correct model of the rabbit heart which he developed in Natalia Trayanova's laboratory[16] based on data from Vetter & McCulloch.[22] This passive bidomain model predicted three-dimensional pattern of VEP, produced by external defibrillation shock (see Figure 7), which were in complete agreement with experimental findings. In addition, it extended experimentally obtained maps to three dimensions. Analysis of shock-induced VEP and post-shock electrical activity revealed that similar to ICD defibrillation, external monophasic shocks are also likely to induce virtual electrode induced phase singularity and arrhythmia.

Thus, we conclude that virtual electrode polarization is a universal mechanism responsible for various modes of defibrillation.

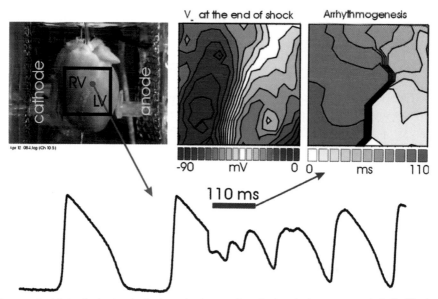

Figure 6. Virtual electrode induced phase singularity during external defibrillation shock.[16] Panels show: photograph of the heart and electrodes, transmembrane voltage distribution at the end of shock, isochronal map of post-shock activation, optical recording from a representative site.

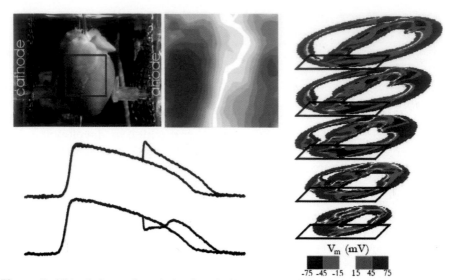

Figure 7. Virtual electrode polarization during external defibrillation shocks. Left: experimental data obtained with optical mapping of a Langendorff-perfused rabbit heart, stained with voltage-sensitive dye. Panels show: photograph of the heart and electrodes, map of VEP, recorded from a field of view shown in the photo, examples of traces recorded from positive and negative polarization areas, superimposed with control traces. Right: Passive bidomain model predictions. Shock-induced polarizations are shown. Electrode configuration reproduced that used in the experiment.

Conclusions

Our findings indicate that electric stimulation of the myocardium produces virtual electrode polarization, consisting of both positive and negative polarization. VEP depends on the strength of the shock, its waveform and electrode configuration. Outcome of pacing or defibrillation stimulus depends on pre-shock phase of electrical activity and electrotonic interaction of areas of opposite polarization. Such interaction may produce break excitation wavefronts, which are responsible for heartbeat initiation during pacing or reentry onset during vulnerability and defibrillation failure. VEP theory provided mechanistic explanation of stimulation of the heart.[15]

References

1. Swammerdam J. **Biblia Naturae**. 1738. H.Boerhaave, Leyden.
2. Galvani L. **De vibribus electricitatis in motu musculari. Commentarius.** De Bononiesi Scientarium et Ertium Instituto atque Academia Commentarii 1791;7:363–416.

3. Hoffa M, Ludwig C. Einige neue Versuche uber Herzbewegung. *Zeitschrift Rationelle Medizin* 1850;9:107–144.
4. Vulpian A. Note sur les effets de la faradisation directe des ventricules du coeur le chien. *Arch de Physiol* 1874; i:975.
5. Prevost JL, Battelli F. Sur quelques effets des decharges electriques sur le coeur mammiferes. *Comptes Rendus Seances Acad Sci* 1899;129:1267.
6. Furman S, Schwedel JB. An intracardiac pacemaker for Stokes-Adams seizures. *N Engl J Med* 1959;261:943–948.
7. Beck CS, Pritchard WH, Feil HS. Ventricular fibrillation of long duration abolished by electric shock. *JAMA* 1947;135:985.
8. Wiggers CJ, Wegria R. Ventricular fibrillation due to single localized induction in condenser shock supplied during the vulnerable phase of ventricular systole. *Am J Physiol* 1939;128:500.
9. Dillon SM. Optical recordings in the rabbit heart show that defibrillation strength shocks prolong the duration of depolarization and the refractory period. *Circ Res* 1991;69:842–856.
10. Davila HV, Salzberg BM, Cohen LB, et al. A large change in axon fluorescence that provides a promising method for measuring membrane potential. *Nat New Biol* 1973;241:159–160.
11. Rattay F. Ways to approximate current-distance relations for electrically stimulated fibers [published erratum appears in J Theor Biol 1987 Oct 21;128(4): 527]. *J Theor Biol* 4-7-1987;125:339–349.
12. Sepulveda NG, Roth BJ, Wikswo JP. Current injection into a two-dimensional anisotropic bidomain. *Biophys J* 1989;55:987–999.
13. Sobie EA, Susil RC, Tung L. A generalized activating function for predicting virtual electrodes in cardiac tissue. *Biophys J* 1997;73:1410–1423.
14. Wikswo JP, Lin S-F, Abbas RA. Virtual electrodes in cardiac tissue: A common mechanism for anodal and cathodal stimulation. *Biophys J* 1995;69:2195–2210.
15. Efimov IR, Gray RA, Roth BJ. Virtual electrodes and de-excitation: New insights into fibrillation induction and defibrillation. *J Cardiovasc Electrophysiol* 2000;11:339–353.
16. Efimov IR, Aguel F, Cheng Y, et al. Virtual electrode polarization in the far field: Implications for external defibrillation. *Am J Physiol* 2000;279:H1055–H1070.
17. Knisley SB, Hill BC, Ideker RE. Virtual electrode effects in myocardial fibers. *Biophys J* 1994;66:719–728.
18. Neunlist M, Tung L. Spatial distribution of cardiac transmembrane potentials around an extracellular electrode: Dependence on fiber orientation. *Biophys J* 1995;68:2310–2322.
19. Nikolski V, Efimov IR. Virtual electrode polarization of ventricular epicardium during bipolar stimulation. *J Cardiovasc Electrophysiol* 2000;11:605.
20. Weidmann S. Effect of current flow on the membrane potential of cardiac muscle. *J Physiol* 1951;115:227–236.
21. Efimov IR, Cheng Y, Van Wagoner DR, et al. Virtual electrode-induced phase singularity: A basic mechanism of failure to defibrillate. *Circ Res* 1998; 82:918–925.
22. Vetter FJ, McCulloch AD. Three-dimensional analysis of regional cardiac function: A model of rabbit ventricular anatomy. *Prog Biophys Mol Biol* 1998;69:157–183.

Part VII.

Discussion: Can Computer Simulations be Useful for the Development of New Therapeutic Strategies?

Chapter 21

Arrhythmia: A Therapeutic Dilemma

Lukas Kappenberger, MD

The clinician finds himself in the center of a triangle with links to physiology, to pathology and to clinical observations, but indeed today there is not much evidence of interconnection of these fields. Moreover, therapeutic interventions are based mainly on empiricism, at least as far as the treatment of arrhythmia is concerned.

To give a more detailed example of this complex situation let us review the milestones in **research** for fibrillation. In 1874 Vulpian[1] described faradization as a possibility to get control over cardiac rhythm. The concept of reentry that was later developed increased our understanding on "Delirium Cordis" and in 1962 Moe already constructed the first computer model upon which basis he hypothesized that a wavefront might fractionate to give offsprings and multiple wavelets, which in turn became the basis for modern understanding of atrial fibrillation.[2]

In contrast to these milestones discoveries, the **treatment** of fibrillation has a completely different and mostly empiric history. In 1749, Senac introduced Quinidine for the treatment of irregular pulse, and in 1959 Lown[3] applied synchronized cardioversion based on custom built defibrillators used to treat cardiac arrest during open-heart surgery. Since this breakthrough in cardiothoracic surgery, there have only been minor developments in therapeutical concepts.

The era of ablation started by accident with the His-bundle being fulgurated while the patient had a defibrillation with a right ventricular catheter in situ. This observation opened the field for in vivo dissection of conductive tissue. It culminates today with a boom in the interventional industry with radiofrequency ablation. However, the interventions are

From Virag N, Blanc O, Kappenberger L (eds): *Computer Simulation and Experimental Assessment of Cardiac Electrophysiology.* ©Futura Publishing Co., Inc., Armonk, NY, 2001.

generally based on empirical considerations rather than on documented physiologic, anatomic or functional substrates.

It is therefore evident that within the field of our interest, therapeutic developments have not always followed the lessons from basic research. Therefore an integration of clinical and research progresses has to be made, and one tool that can offer us this possibility is the computer. In fact we might only be at the very beginning of the use of artificial intelligence and computer power for the study of life sciences. There is however good hope that this new tool will allow further growth of our knowledge. This idea is based on observation of history. Developments and science can only progress if there is intensive communication between researchers. This communication needs a transmitter medium which apparently was the limiting factor if one goes back in history. Figure 1 shows that there was a clear stagnation of knowledge in medieval times until about 1500 when Gutenberg invented the art of printing. As a result of this development, texts did not have to be written by hand anymore. This invention clearly led to a nearly unlimited outspread of knowledge until the mid-eighties of the 20th century when it was no longer possible to print all the important new knowledge on paper. For the field of medicine alone, the annual printed material would fill a bookshelf of 1.5 km. Computer is the tool that allowed to further document knowledge, create the needed contacts for exchange of ideas and thereby increase the scientific knowledge of the community.

Now we will encounter the genetic limitations of our brain capacity. The accumulation of knowledge by an individual in order to synthesize a new idea is possibly limited. Artificial aids could enlarge knowledge and

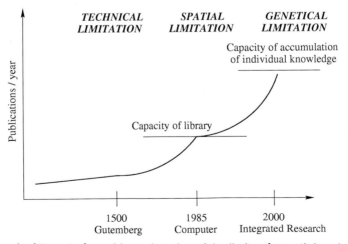

Figure 1. Attempt of graphic explanation of the limits of growth in science.

computer simulation may allow the creation of a virtual environment where human fantasy, which is hopefully unlimited, can continue to develop. We therefore believe that integrated research with computer simulation will make it possible to perform virtual experiments, and virtual interventions leading to new and better therapies for diseased patients. Such concepts and chains of developments are, of course, not new; in the aeronautical industry for example, computer power assists the development of aerodynamical and structural concepts. Today learning to fly the most complex airplanes would not be possible without computer assistance, and we accept that simulator training is an essential part of reliable airplane flying.

Why not apply this concept then to the development of new medical solutions? We anticipate that computer simulation can be used to answer how geometry and anatomy can influence electrical stability in a heart structure. It should also be possible to define the critical mass of tissue for initiation, maintenance or exhaustion of arrhythmic events. There is increasing evidence that the electrophysiological background is not a stable system but that it underlies oscillations like any biological system. Such fluctuations of the background can be simulated and their impact studied in a way that would not be possible in an animal model. Furthermore, the study of the effect of selected membrane channels on the tissue or organ function is very difficult in biologic experiments today. In this context, some antiarrhythmic therapies are classical examples of misinterpretation of basic research. For example, the classification of antiarrhythmic agents according to Vaughan Williams, studied by generations of medical students, describes phenomena happening on the cellular level but not in the organ. As a result of this, progresses in the pharmacological control of arrhythmias have been slower. Such misinterpretations should be prevented and computer assisted research could hopefully be one way to achieve this objective. One major difficulty in the whole field of living sciences is the different scales involved. This is particularly true in cardiac arrhythmia, both in space (from proteins, to cells, and to whole organs) and in time (from milliseconds to whole human life). The link between these scales remains challenging from an experimental point of view. Computer simulations could give us access to such different scales and help us to bridge them.

Our aim is to integrate basic electrophysiological research and biological experiments in order to develop new pharmacological, electrical or surgical therapeutic strategies. Promising solutions are at the doorstep, as evidenced in many chapters of this book. Furthermore, the development of computer hardware and software is so rapid that it is hard to estimate today where this technique will bring us in five years. On the other hand computer experiments will not be contaminated by factors that are not under control. Whether this will be an advantage or on the contrary a limitation, due to the absence of spontaneity, remains to be established. Naturally, as everywhere, there are limitations to take into consideration and a computer model will not be more perfect than any other experiment, but it has the power to make a better synthesis of our knowledge than conventional biological experiments, which in any case must continue.

With computer simulations the following questions arise. How much ignorance can we accept? How much irrealism can we accept? How much detail is needed to come to new conclusions, meaning how much information must be integrated in the model? Finally, as in every field of human activity, how much time can we invest, which in this case means how much calculation power is needed? Such reflections hold true for every experiment where each step away from reality is a compromise, and every model allows just a look at a specific part of a problem. But after all, how can we understand reality other than thinking in models?

References

1. Vulpian A. Note sur les effets de la faradisation directe des ventricules du cœur du chien. *Arch de Physiol* 1874;975.
2. Moe G. On the multiple wavelets hypothesis of atrial fibrillation. *Arch Int Pharmacodyn Ther* 1962;140:183–188.
3. Lown B, Amarasingham R, Neuman J. New method for terminating cardiac arrhythmias: Use of synchronized capacitor discharge. Electric cardioversion of atrial fibrillation. *JAMA* 1962;182:548–555.

Index